OPERATIVE

PROCEDURE

Published by
ETHICON, INC.
Somerville, New Jersey

TABLE OF CONTENTS

TABLE OF CONTENTS (Continued)

FOREWORD

AMERICAN SURGERY has made great strides in the last decade. In few branches of science has advancement been so dynamic and so accelerated. To keep pace with this ever-changing cavalcade of surgical progress, the publishers of Operative Procedure have made numerous revisions in the previous eight editions, which were prepared in collaboration with the staff of *Surgery, Gynecology & Obstetrics.*

The ninth edition has been completely revised and edited with the cooperation of a board of outstanding surgeons. Each subject to be illustrated has been carefully selected and presented in a step-by-step manner. To aid in clarification and orientation, descriptive text accompanies each drawing.

Most of the drawings in this book are adapted from original work drawn for the previous editions by Messrs. W. C. Shepard and Tom Jones, to whom grateful acknowledgement is made.

Many new operations have been added, and a number of procedures have been deleted because of obsolescence. An entirely new section on Traumatic and War Surgery has been incorporated.

To the surgeons who, by their contributions to the science of surgery, made this publication possible, we acknowledge a deep and sincere debt of gratitude.

To the student, to the teacher, to the practicing surgeon both in civil life and with our armed forces, we hope that this latest edition of Operative Procedure will prove both informative and useful.

TWO-HAND KNOT TIE
(AFTER PARTIPILO)

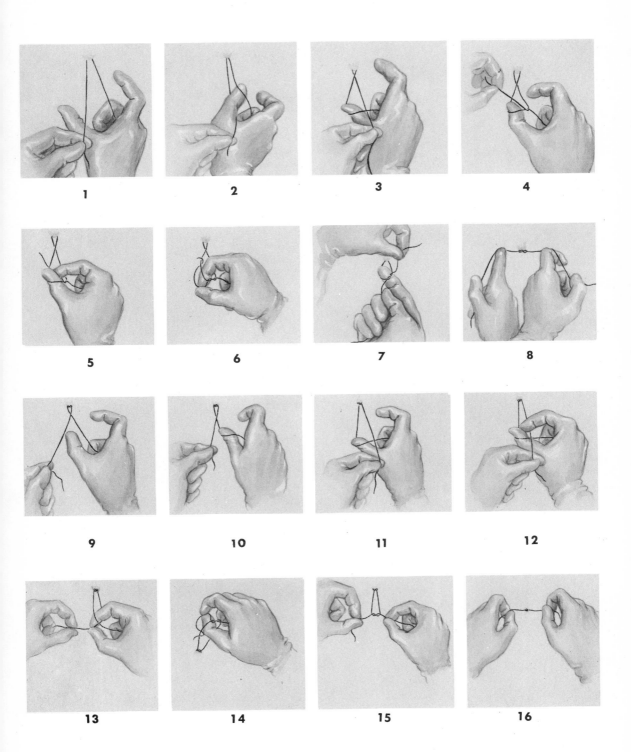

1

2

3

4

5

6

7

8

9

10

11

12

13

14

15

16

NOTE: The two-hand square knot illustrated
may be begun with either the right or left hand.

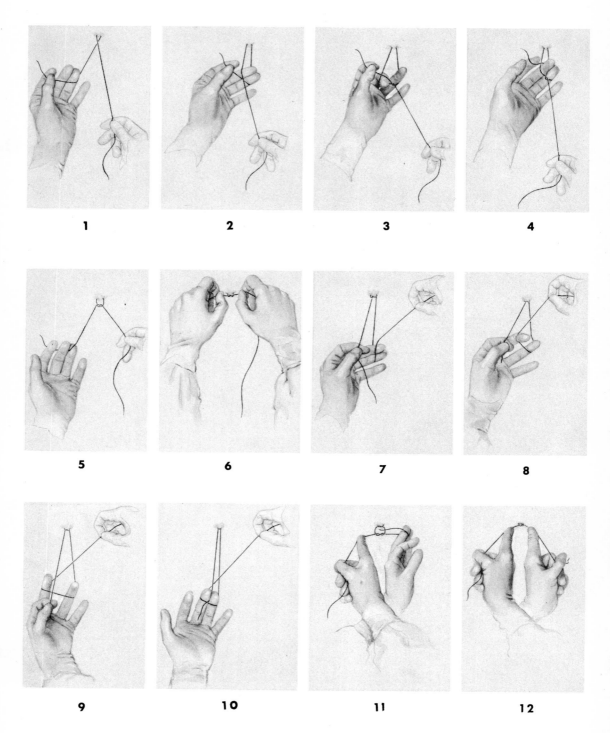

NOTE: Shown here is the left hand beginning the knot with the short end of the ligature. However, either hand may be used in this initial step.

TECHNIQUE OF INSTRUMENT TIE
(MURPHY)

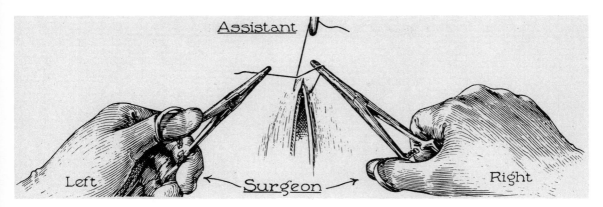

1. The short end of the suture is held taut by the assistant's forceps shown in upper margin. The surgeon holds the long end of the suture in his left forceps and utilizes the right forceps to form the loop.

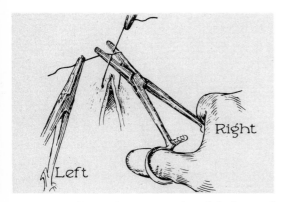

2. The right forceps is now opened, and the long end of the suture grasped as the left forceps is removed.

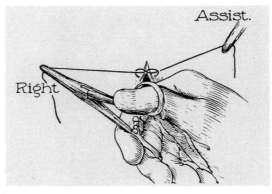

3. First half-hitch is accomplished by the surgeon's forceps moved to right and the assistant's to left.

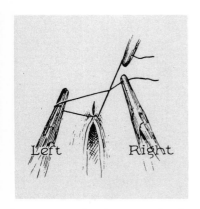

4. First knot has been completed. Second square knot begun.

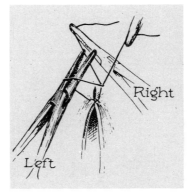

5. Similar procedure to Fig. 3. Loop is made with the left forceps.

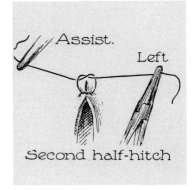

6. Second half-hitch completed by crossing over from right to left.

TECHNIQUE OF PLACING DEEP LIGATURES
(PRINTY, GRANT)

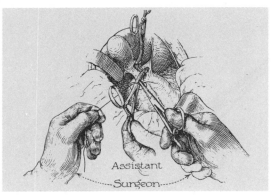

1. First half-hitch is taken loosely and slipped down over the tip of holding forceps.

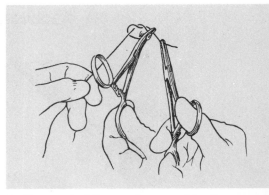

2. Short end of ligature is grasped by forceps and the ligature tightened around pedicle.

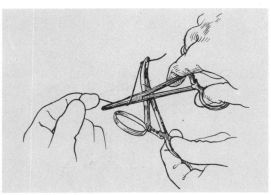

3. A second half-hitch is begun by looping long end around forceps in the right hand.

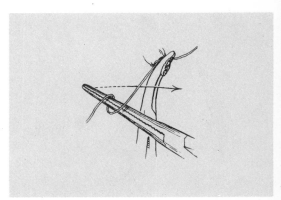

4. Method of beginning second half-hitch by looping around forceps. Holding forceps left in place.

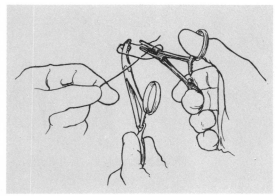

5. After loop is thrown around forceps, short end is grasped by opening forceps and pulled through.

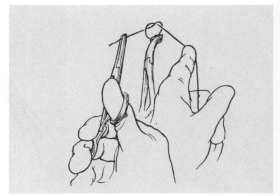

6. Second half-hitch completed by crossing hands. This method is helpful in regions difficult of access.

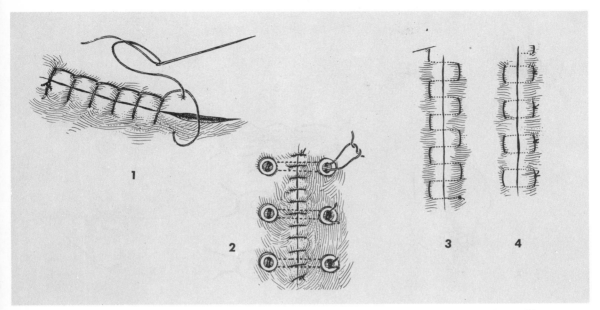

1. The blanket or continuous locked suture. **2.** Continuous suture and method of using perforated buttons to support tension sutures. **3.** Continuous mattress suture. **4.** Interrupted mattress suture.

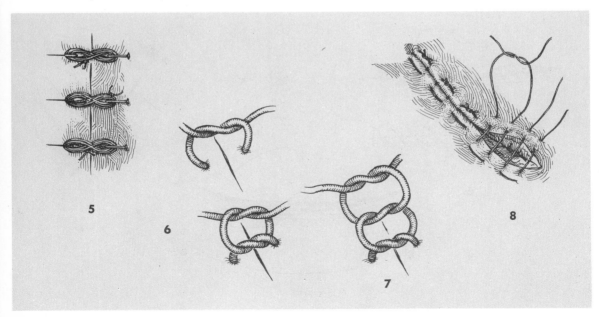

5. Figure-of-eight tension sutures around pins. **6.** Method of placing first and second half-hitches in the square or true knot. **7.** The square knot reinforced by third half-hitch. **8.** The Halsted interrupted mattress suture.

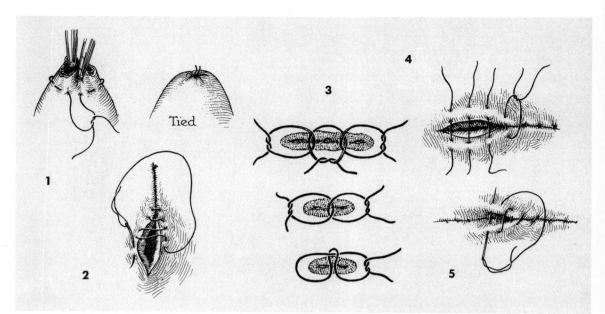

1. Purse-string suture around open stump. **2.** Closing stump by Cushing stitch. **3.** Methods for ligation of pedicles with anchored ligatures. **4.** Interrupted Lembert inverting stitch. **5.** Continuous Lembert stitch.

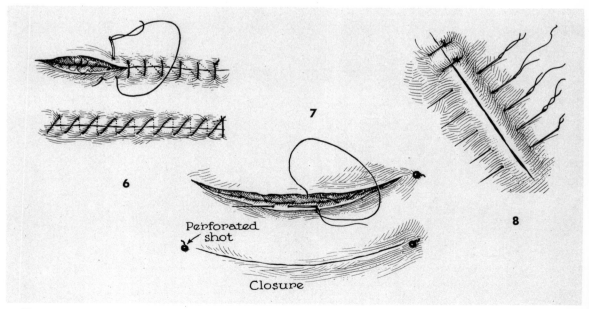

6. Two methods of continuous over-and-over closing sutures. **7.** Subcuticular suture for closure of skin incision. Perforated buck shot used to anchor suture. **8.** Interrupted skin sutures—multiple needle technique.

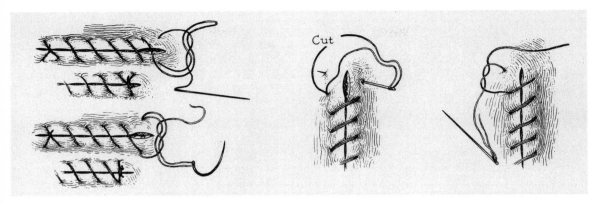

1. Variety of methods for securing the ends of completed continuous sutures. Technique for securing ends of both double and single sutures is demonstrated. Note method of dividing suture to avoid double thickness of knot.

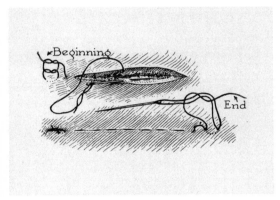

2. Method of beginning subcuticular suture by placing square knot lateral to incision. Method of ending suture at opposite end of incision.

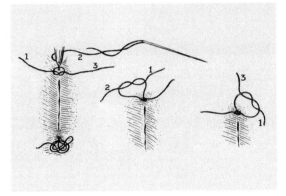

3. Alternate method for the completion of subcuticular continuous suture by placing a holding knot around end of subcuticular suture.

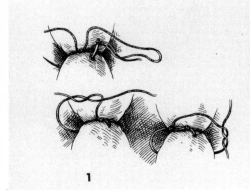

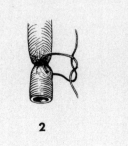

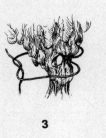

4. Methods of placing transfixing ligatures to prevent slipping. (1) Transfixing ligature of pedicle. (2) Method of placing transfixing ligature in vessel. (3) Tying transfixing ligature of omentum or of hernial sac.

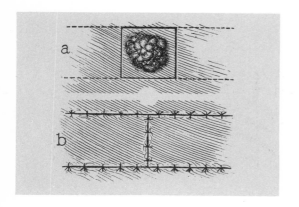
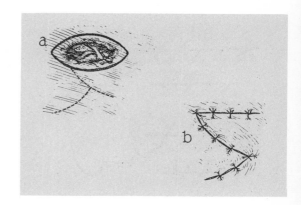
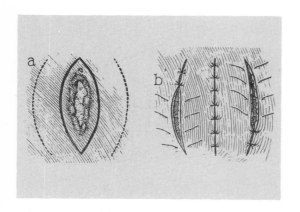
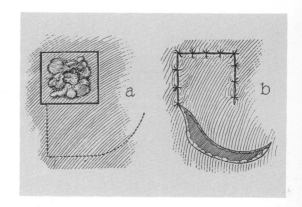
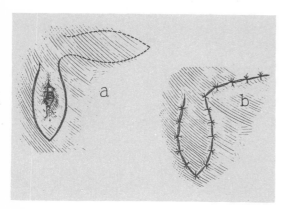
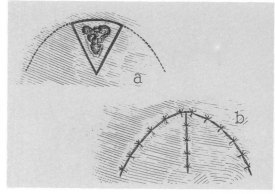

Illustrated here are a number of examples of sliding full-thickness flaps used to fill wide skin defects. The choice of procedure is dependent upon the size, shape, and location of the defect.

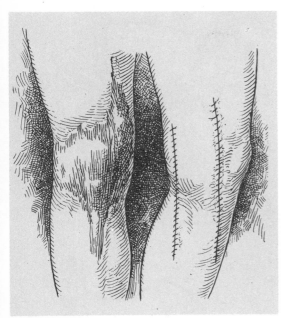

1. Burn contracture over anterior surface of knee. Flap raised from opposite leg and sutured in its bed.

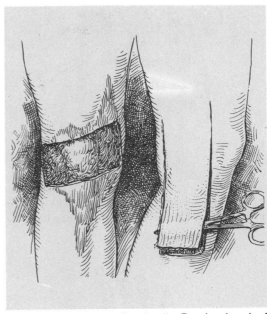

2. Scar tissue excised over patella. Previously raised flap on opposite leg held and ready for transfer.

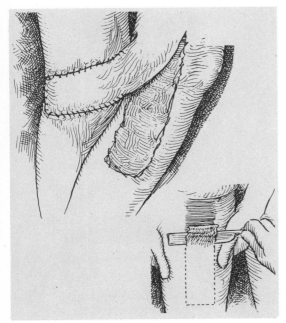

3. Flap sutured. Raw surface left by elevation of graft covered by Tiersch graft. Insert shows Tiersch graft.

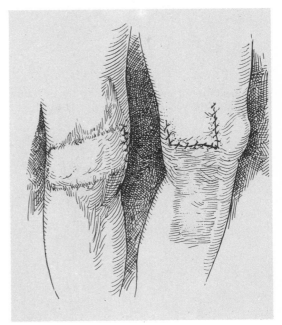

4. End result after division of flap from opposite leg. Covering completed of remaining raw surface.

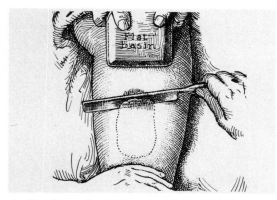

1. Cutting split thickness graft from thigh—skin under tension (Padgett Dermatome may be used).

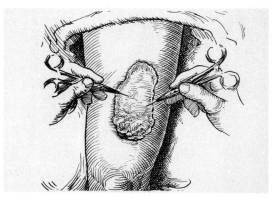

2. Site of graft has been prepared. Split thickness graft is teased into correct position with needles.

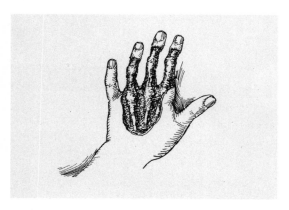

3. Appearance of granulation bed after excision of scar tissue following burn contracture of hand.

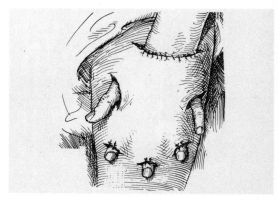

4. Method of obtaining full thickness graft by placing hand in pocket flap on anterior surface of thigh.

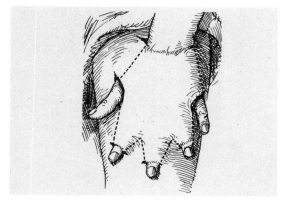

5. After a period of several days, the flap is divided by multiple incisions indicated by dotted lines.

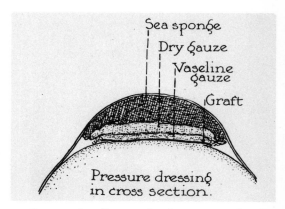

Sea sponge
Dry gauze
Vaseline gauze
Graft

Pressure dressing in cross section.

6. Cross section diagram showing pressure dressing frequently utilized following most skin grafts.

SURGICAL TREATMENT OF PENETRATING
WOUNDS OF THE ABDOMEN

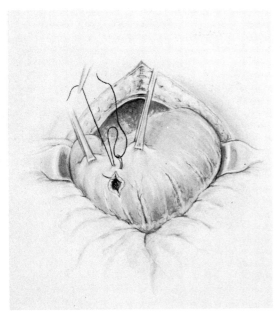

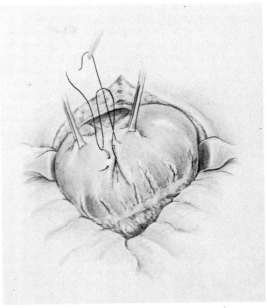

1. Lacerated edges of debrided wound. Defect closed transversely by Connell inverting suture.

2. Second row of Connell inverting sutures. Similar technique is used in repair of perforated peptic ulcers.

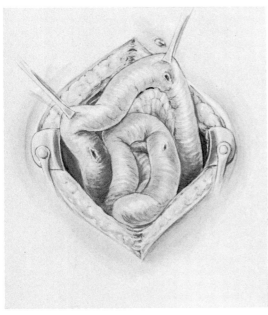

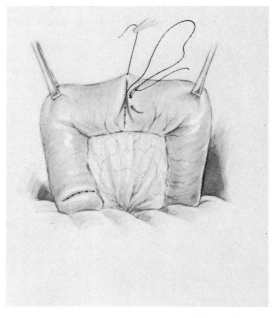

3. Multiple penetrating wounds of small intestine. If blood supply is impaired, resection is indicated.

4. Method of repair by two rows of inverting sutures. Closure always made in transverse diameter.

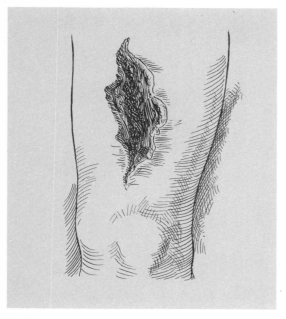

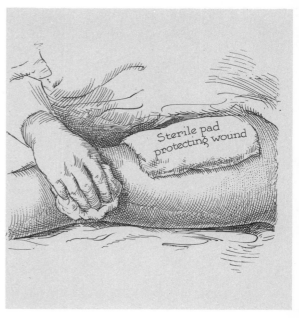

1. Recent lacerated wound of thigh involving skin, fascia and underlying muscle. No fracture of femur.

2. Wide skin area thoroughly cleansed. Cotton pledgets preferable to gauze or other rough material.

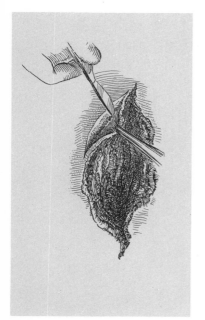

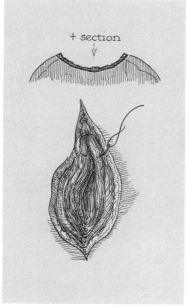

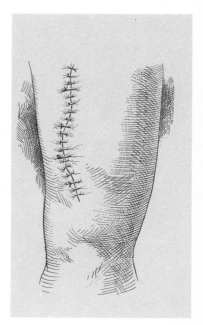

3. Debridement of wound margins. Sulfonamide may be applied.

4. Approximation of edges by interrupted, widely placed sutures.

5. Primary closure of defect by interrupted, widely placed sutures.

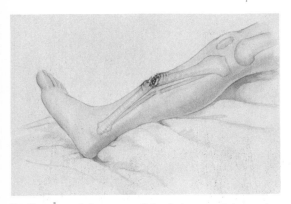

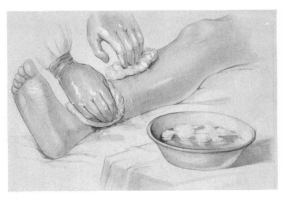

1. Compound fracture of both bones of lower leg showing laceration of skin on the anterior surface.

2. Leg placed on sterile sheets, wound protected by means of sterile gauze. Skin is thoroughly cleansed.

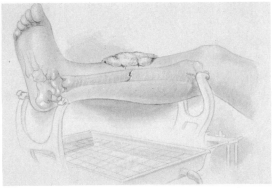

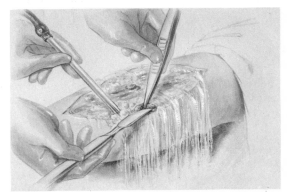

3. Fractured ends of tibia debrided. Aligned by bone pins and traction apparatus. Note pan under leg.

4. Thorough debridement under stream of sterile saline solution, facilitating removal of loose particles.

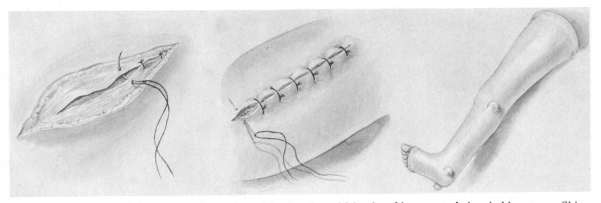

5. Beginning closure of clean edges of muscle and fascia using widely placed interrupted absorbable sutures. Skin closure by widely placed interrupted non-absorbable sutures. Full-length plaster cast in which pins are incorporated, extends from toes to groin and permits early ambulation. (Note: This method is usually applicable only to compound fractures less than eight hours old. No sutures used under combat conditions.)

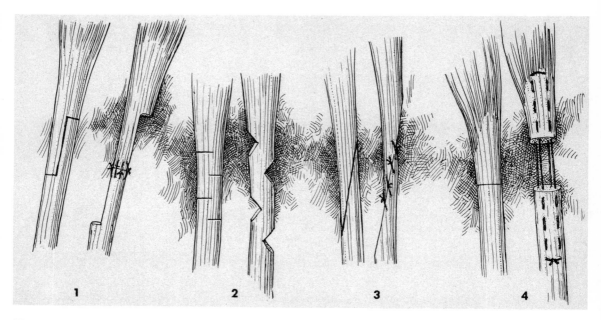

Transverse methods of tendon lengthening and repair. **1.** Half section slitting and gliding ("Z" tenotomy) method. **2.** Accordion method. **3.** Oblique section and gliding method. **4.** Lange method.

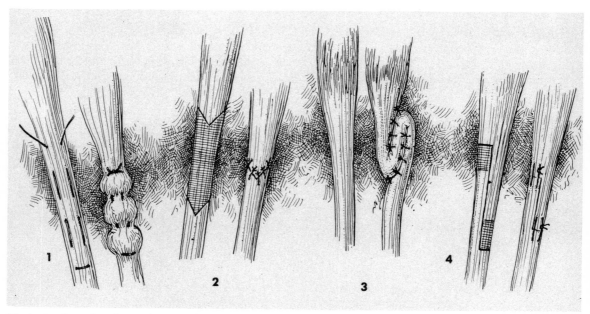

Methods of tendon shortening. **1.** Hoffa's method. **2.** Removal of section of tendon and mortise. Method of uniting ends. **3.** Doubling over method and technique of suturing folds. **4.** "Z" incision with excision of ends.

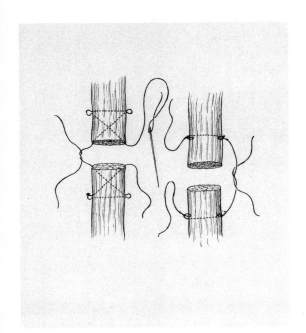

Placing tension sutures in divided tendons. Dotted lines indicate sutures passing through tendons.

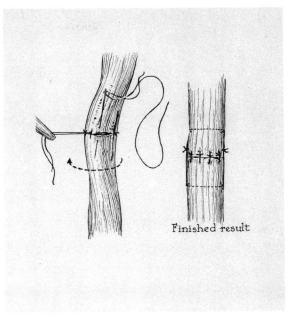

Tension suture utilized for rotation to permit introduction of additional sutures for accurate coaptation.

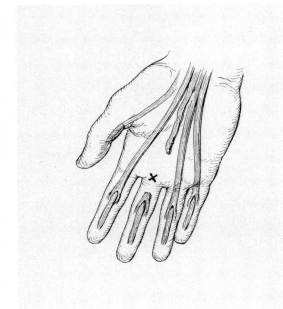

Common site (X) of tendon laceration in hand. Marked retraction of proximal and distal tendon ends.

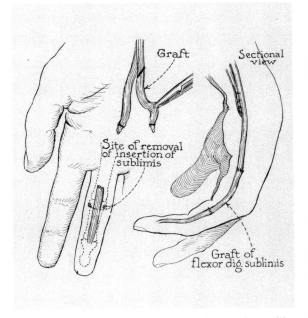

Repair of flexor digitorum profundus tendon utilizing tendon graft from flexor digitorum sublimis.

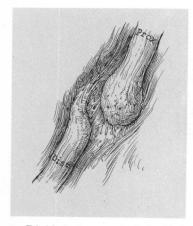

1. Divided nerve ends imbedded in scar tissue. Note neuroma.

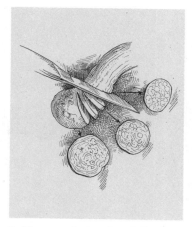

2. Neuroma isolated and sliced until normal funiculi are reached.

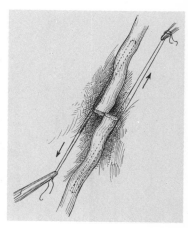

3. Guy sutures placed in sheath on posterior aspect of nerve.

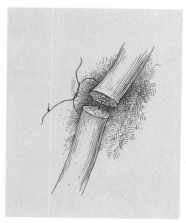

4. Approximating suture placed at midpoint of posterior surface.

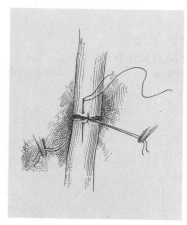

5. Approximating suture placed at midpoint of anterior surface.

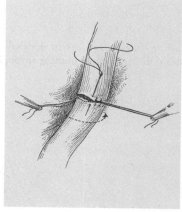

6. Successive sutures placed in neural sheath as nerve is rotated.

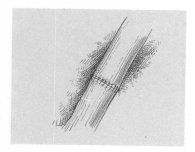

7. Completed suture. Showing approximation of neural sheath.

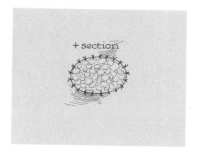

8. Diagrammatic cross section showing sutures in neural sheath.

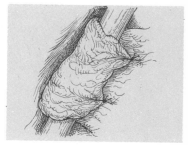

9. Optional method of protecting suture line with flap of fat.

REPAIR OF WOUNDS OF THE HEART

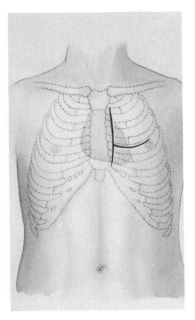

1. Anatomical relations. "T" incision and wide exposure of left heart.

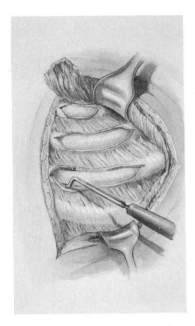

2. Incision of periosteum and freeing of ribs with rib dissector.

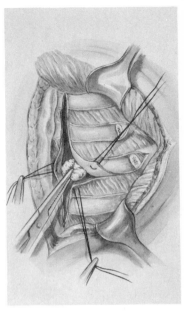

3. Pericardium held with three guy sutures and "T" incision made.

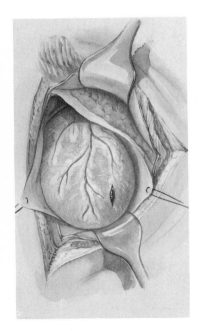

4. Exposure of left heart. Visualization of wound of myocardium.

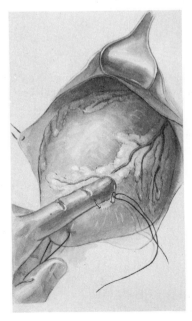

5. Digital control of bleeding while sutures of gut are placed.

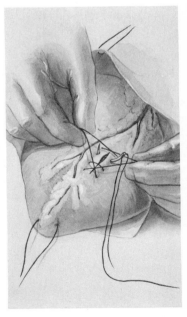

6. Tightening of suture. Note guy suture placed in apex of heart.

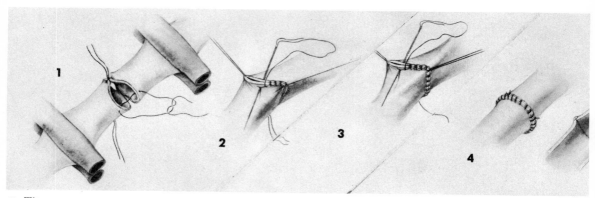

1. Three guy sutures placed equidistant to be used as sutures in final step. **2.** Method of placing continuous suture. **3.** Continuation of suture as vessel is rotated by means of guy sutures. **4.** Suture completed.

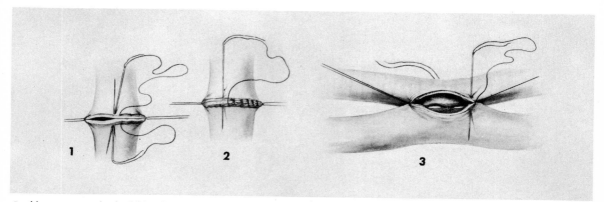

1. Alternate method of blood vessel anastomosis using continuous cobbler's stitch. **2.** Guy sutures used to rotate vessel. **3.** Lateral anastomosis of vessel carrying out triangulation of suture line by guy sutures.

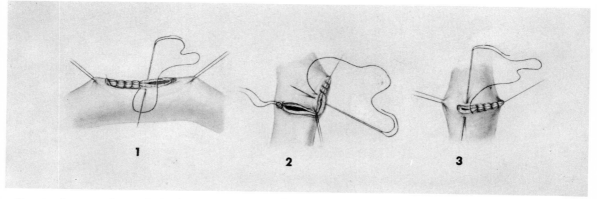

Repair of cuts and tears in blood vessels. **1.** Continuous lock stitch to repair longitudinal tear. **2.** Repair of irregular tear utilizing guy sutures at angles. **3.** Repair of transverse tear by continuous suture.

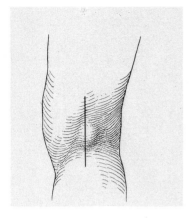

1. Incision for operation on aneurysm of popliteal artery.

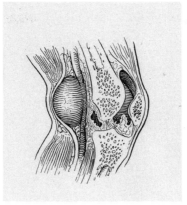

2. Diagrammatic sagittal section showing location of aneurysmal sac.

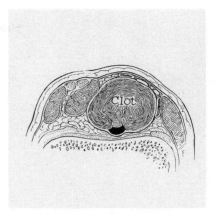

3. Position of clot in relation to tibial nerve and popliteal vein.

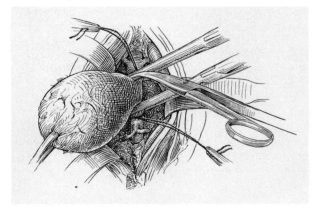

4. Short segment of popliteal artery between ligatures. Sac is removed together with arterial segment.

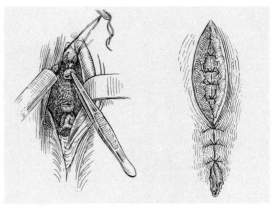

5. Proximal end doubly ligated. Heparin injection optional. Closure by interrupted sutures.

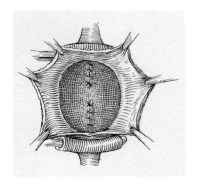

6. Endo-aneurysmorrhaphy, provisional control between clamps.

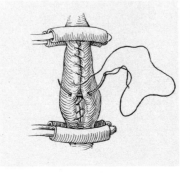

7. Obliterative suture of all openings. Plication of sac wall (Matas).

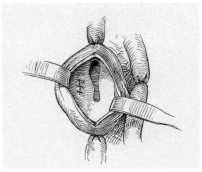

8. Alternate method. Ligatures proximal and distal to sac (Reid).

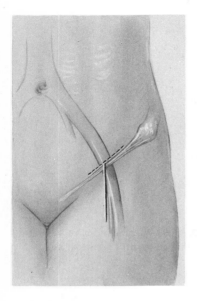

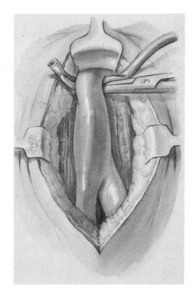

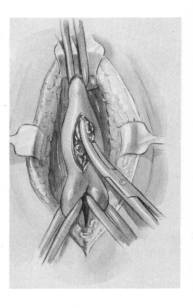

1. Location of incisions for the exposure of femoral or iliac vessels.

2. Exposure of iliac vessel. Catheters inserted for constriction.

3. Tension on catheters. Longitudinal incision and extraction of clot.

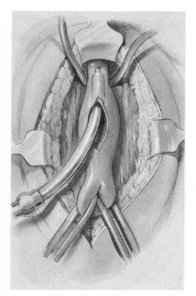

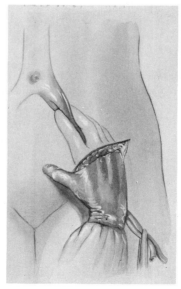

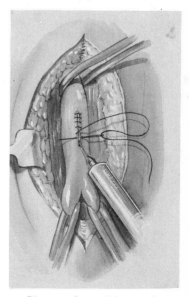

4. Catheters relaxed. Suction tube inserted to extract clot fragments.

5. Milking of common iliac vessel by insertion of hand into incision.

6. Closure of vessel by continuous suture. Injection of heparin.

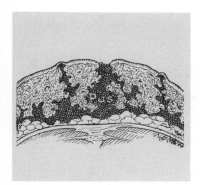

1. Extensive carbuncle, undermining of subcutaneous tissue.

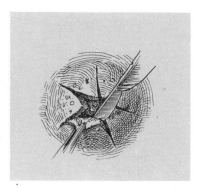

2. Multiple stellate incisions with undercutting of skin flaps.

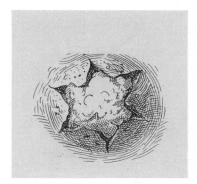

3. Method of placing gauze packing following stellate incisions.

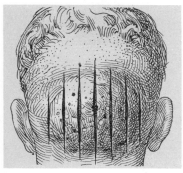

4. Gridiron incisions used only for very extensive carbuncles (Maes).

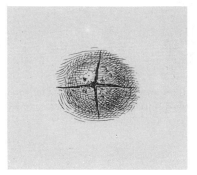

5. Simple crucial incisions for treatment of small carbuncles.

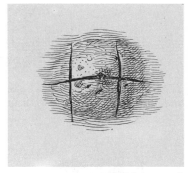

6. Double crucial incisions used for moderate sized carbuncles.

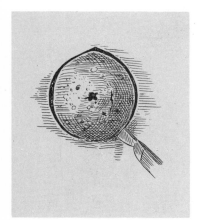

7. Excision of indurated tissue in carbuncle of long standing.

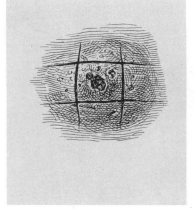

8. Method of excision of necrotic tissue by square-shaped incisions.

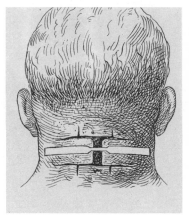

9. Following initial drainage, edges approximated by adhesive.

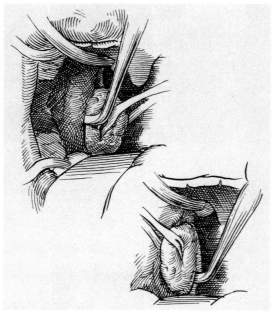

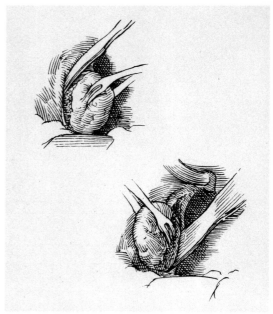

1. Mucous membrane incised along pillars anterior and posterior to tonsil. Tonsil held by tonsil forceps.

2. The tonsil is freed from its fossa by use of dissector and traction on tonsil-holding forceps.

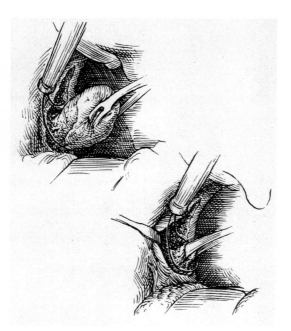

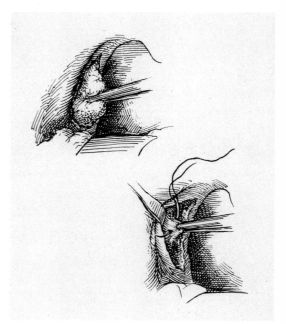

3. Snare applied over special tonsil-holding forceps. Tonsil removed. Tonsil remnants removed by snare.

4. Methods of hemostasis. Pressure by gauze pack or bleeder sutured with fine absorbable catgut.

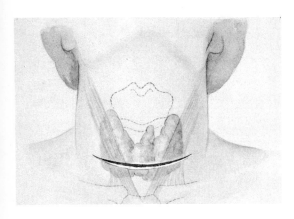

1. Relationship of incision to thyroid gland. Incision passes through skin, fat, and platysma.

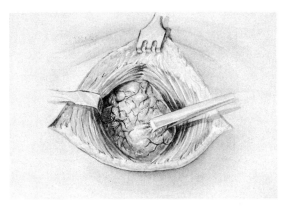

2. Strap muscles separated in midline, lobe elevated, lateral vein ligated.

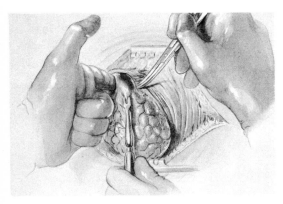

3. Upper pole retracted downward, curved forceps introduced underneath medial side.

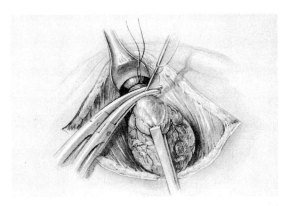

4. Proximal ligature tied. Superior pole is divided between clamps.

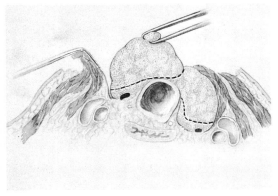

5. Cross section showing retraction of strap muscles and general scheme of resection.

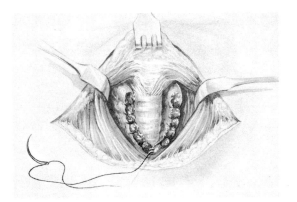

6. Resection completed and remnants sutured. Reconstruction of isthmus to fill sternal hollow.

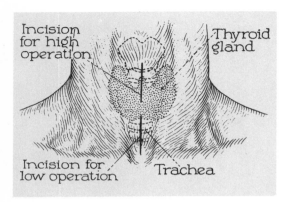

1. Surface anatomy showing relationship of high and low incisions to underlying structures.

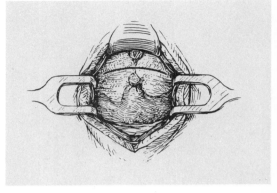

2. Technique of high tracheotomy. The pretracheal fascia is incised at the level of the cricoid cartilage.

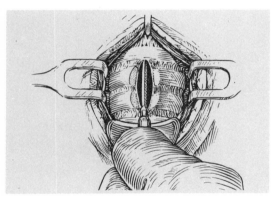

3. Cricoid cartilage retracted to steady trachea. First, second, and third cartilaginous rings incised.

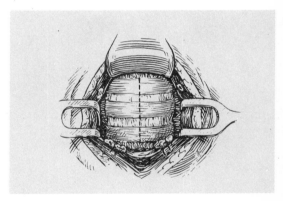

4. Technique of low tracheotomy. Dotted line indicates incision. Low site is inadvisable in children.

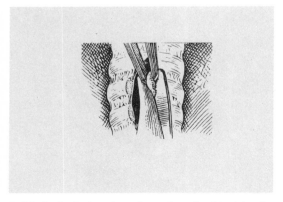

5. Method of trimming edges of tracheal incision in order to establish an oval-shaped opening (Digby).

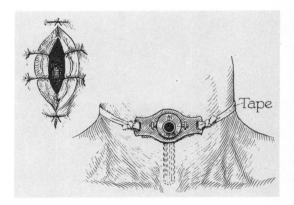

6. Method of fixing trachea by through and through sutures. Method for holding tracheal tube by tape.

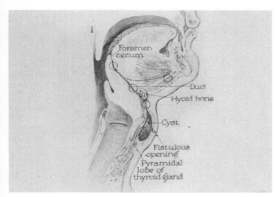

1. Head and neck showing surgical anatomy and location of thyroglossal cyst and duct (Gilman).

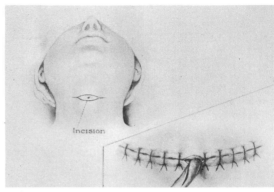

2. Incision around fistula. Insert shows method of closure with drainage after completion of operation.

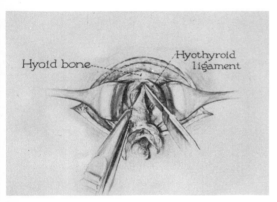

3. Method for complete excision of fistulous tract down to the hyoid bone. Note hyothyroid ligament.

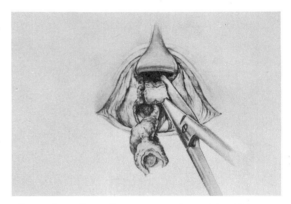

4. Resection of small central portion of hyoid bone through which the fistula passes.

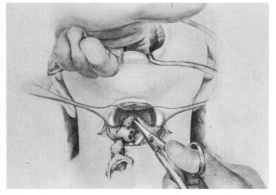

5. Completion of dissection of fistula behind hyoid bone using index finger at base of tongue as guide.

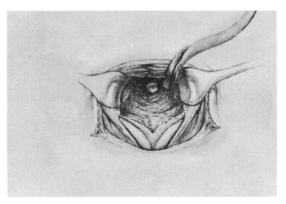

6. Fistula has been completely excised. A Penrose drain is inserted up to the base of the tongue.

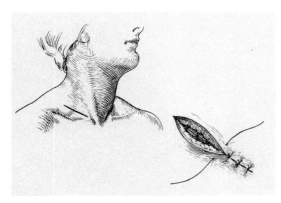

1. Location of incision parallel to and above clavicle is indicated. Insert shows completion of closure.

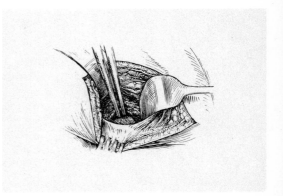

2. Retractors placed, trans-scapular vessels visualized. Vessels doubly clamped for ligation and division.

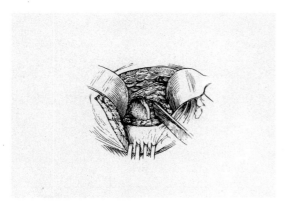

3. Illustration shows method of exposure of phrenic nerve and its relation to scalenus anticus muscle.

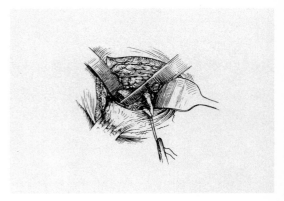

4. Phrenic nerve retracted. Muscle cut transversely releasing compression on subclavian artery.

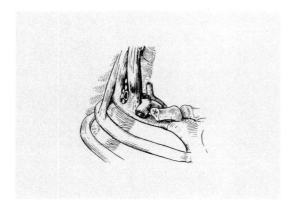

5. Original anatomical defect produced by scalenus anticus muscle pulling up first rib to compress vessel.

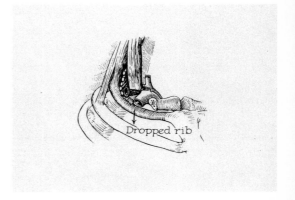

6. Diagram illustrating postoperative result with release of compression of vessel after muscle is cut.

INCISION OF BREAST FOR ABSCESS AND
REMOVAL OF SMALL TUMORS

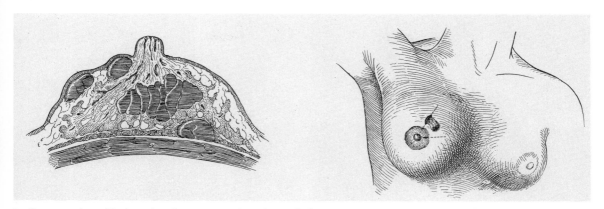

1. Cross section of breast showing common locations of abscesses. Note premammary and retromammary locations. Location of skin incisions radiating from nipple used for superficial lesions, usually without drainage.

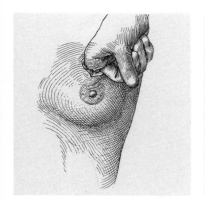

2. Finger introduced to break up fibrous partitions of abscess.

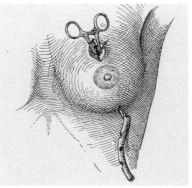

3. Counter incision made on lower aspect of breast for drainage.

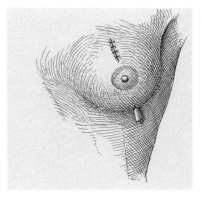

4. Primary incision sutured. Drain still present in counter incision.

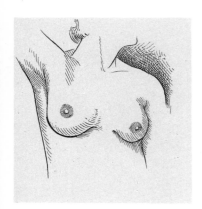

5. Incision in inferior fold for approach to retromammary lesions.

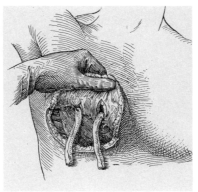

6. Method of placing and anchoring drains in retromammary tissue.

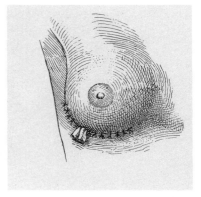

7. Closure of inferior fold incision and placing of soft rubber drains.

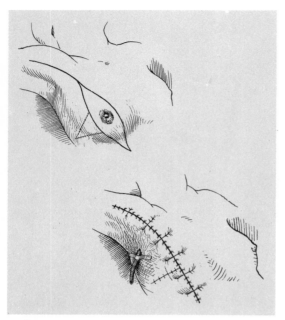

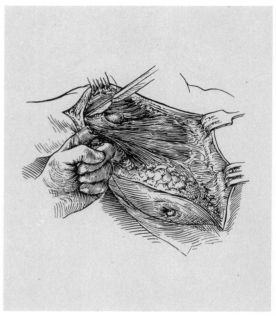

1. Skin incision most commonly employed and optional incision. Lower figure shows closure with drain.

2. Breast retracted exposing pectoralis major muscle. Division of muscle fibres from humeral attachment.

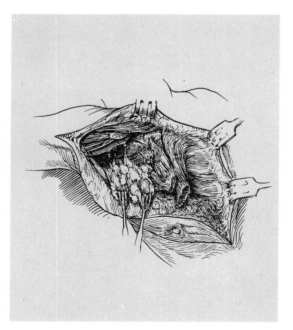

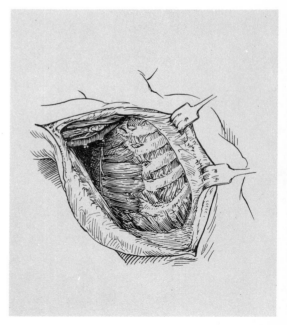

3. Pectoralis minor muscle separated from coracoid attachment. Lymph nodes dissected from axilla.

4. Dissection completed, all axillary nodes resected. All bleeding controlled. Wound ready for closure.

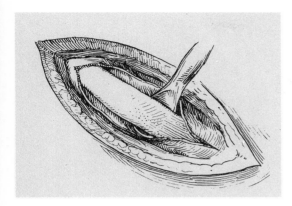

1. Initial step in open method technique. Incision through periosteum and periosteum freed from rib.

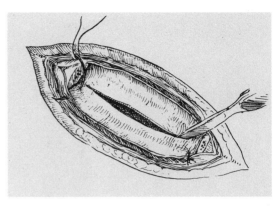

2. Rib has been resected and periosteum anchored. Incision is being made into the pleural cavity.

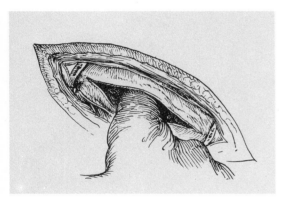

3. The finger is carefully introduced through pleural incision to facilitate removal of fibrinous material.

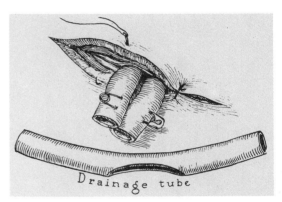

4. Drainage tube bent into "U" and anchored. Skin margins approximated by interrupted sutures.

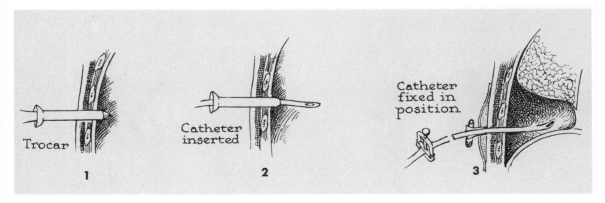

1. Initial step in closed method operation. Trocar inserted into pleural cavity. **2.** A rubber catheter is introduced through the trocar into pleural cavity. **3.** Trocar removed and catheter fixed in empyema cavity.

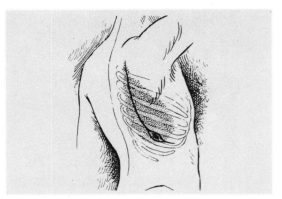

1. Surface anatomy and location of incision which includes fistulous opening. Note extent of cavity.

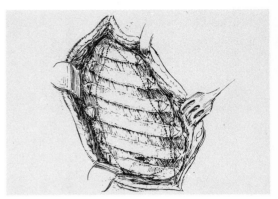

2. Six ribs have been resected. Area of thickened pleura to be removed is indicated by dotted line.

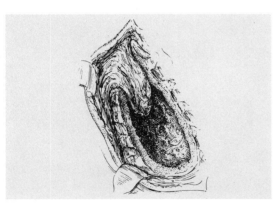

3. Cavity is completely exposed. Method of using muscle flap to cover site of fistulae is shown.

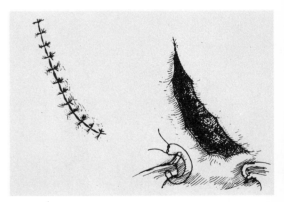

4. Methods of closure. Wound may be completely closed or left open with the skin margins inverted.

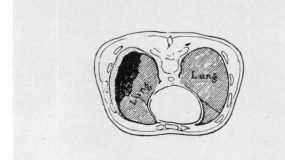

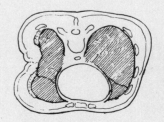

5. Diagrammatic cross section of chest at level of empyema cavity prior to operation. **6.** Cross section of chest at same level after operation demonstrating the complete obliteration of the cavity.

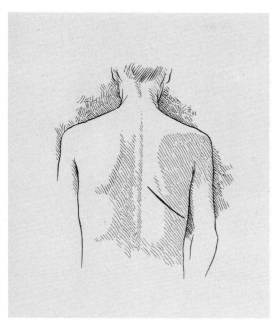

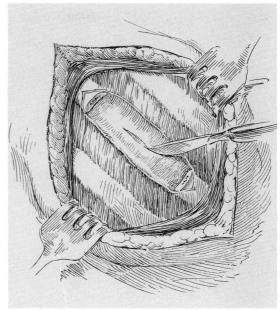

1. Incision is made directly over mid-portion of site of abscess following line of underlying rib.

2. Section of rib excised. Extensive exploratory incision is now made through the periosteal bed.

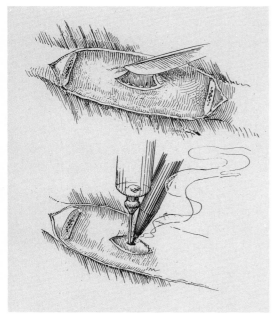

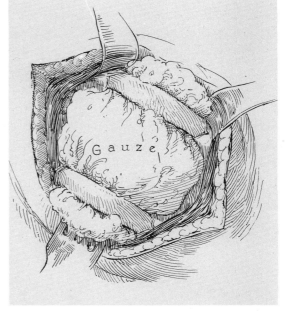

3. Abscess localized by aspiration of pus through incision. Incision into abscess with cautery.

4. Alternate method utilizing two stage operation. Formation of adhesions is induced by gauze pack.

SURGICAL TREATMENT
OF DIAPHRAGMATIC HERNIA

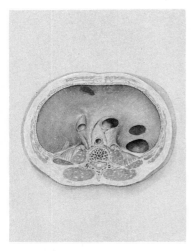

1. Anatomy of diaphragm showing most common sites of herniation.

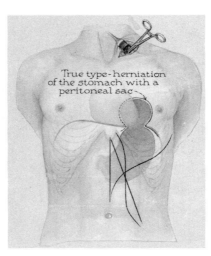

2. Various incisions. Crushing of phrenic nerve precedes operation.

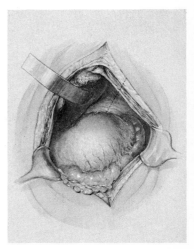

3. Left lobe of liver immobilized by cutting suspensory ligament.

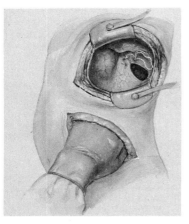

4. Bi-incisional approach. Thoracic approach requires rib resection.

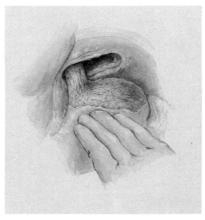

5. Peritoneal sac now separated from stomach (Harrington).

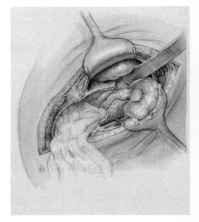

6. Combined incision. Costal cartilages cut, diaphragm divided.

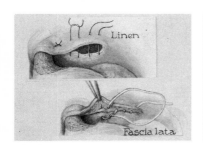

7. Two steps in Harrington method of overlapping closure.

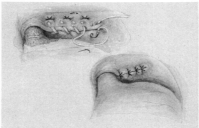

8. Closure continued. Interrupted silk may be used in young children.

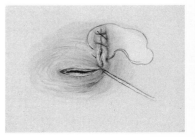

9. Alternative method of closing opening by forming angle.

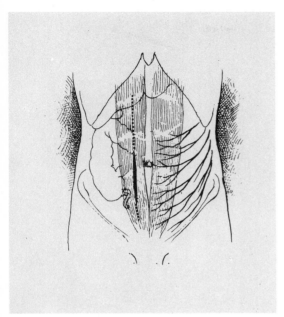

1. Relation of incision to rectus muscle and line for extending incision. Nerve supply to right rectus.

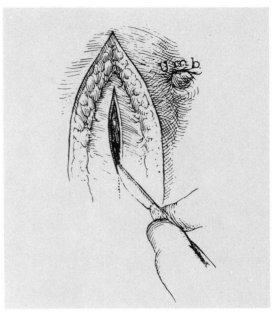

2. Skin and subcutaneous tissue incised. Anterior sheath divided two centimeters lateral to midline.

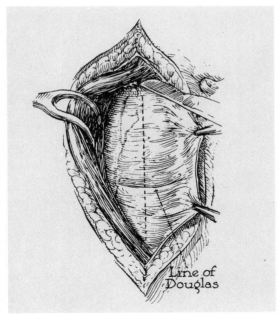

3. Rectus muscle separated in midline, retracted. Posterior rectus sheath and peritoneum exposed.

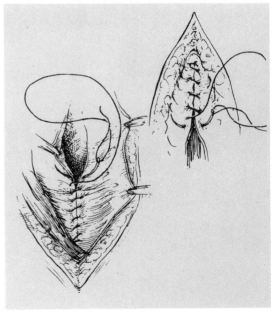

4. Method of closure of posterior rectus sheath and peritoneum. Closure of anterior rectus sheath.

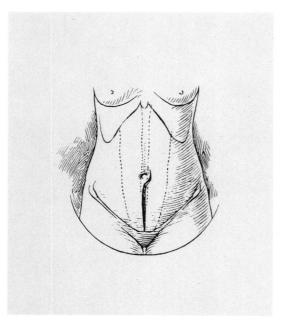

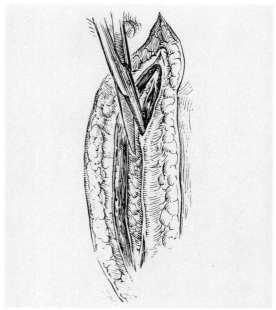

1. Surface anatomy with rectus muscles outlined. Low midline incision between recti muscles.

2. Skin and subcutaneous tissue incised. The anterior rectus sheath is split following the linea alba.

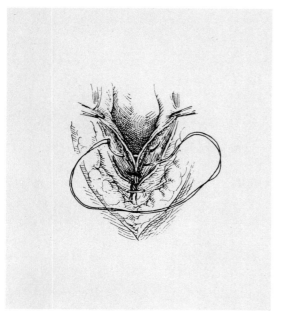

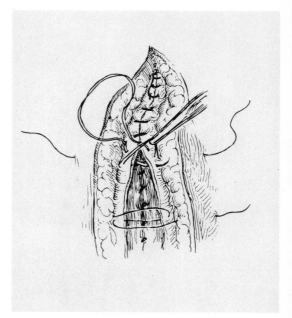

3. Method of closure of the posterior rectus sheath and peritoneum by means of a continuous suture.

4. Through and through tension sutures. Anterior rectus sheath sutured by interrupted technique.

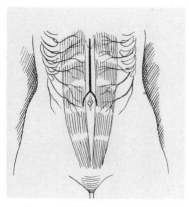

1. Sloan incision showing conservation of nerve supply to rectus.

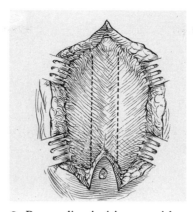

2. Paramedian incisions on either side of midline in rectus sheath.

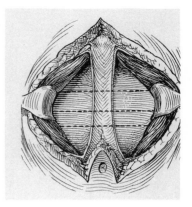

3. Posterior rectus sheath incised transversely at one of three levels.

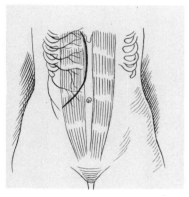

1. Bevan vertical elliptical skin incision conserving nerve supply.

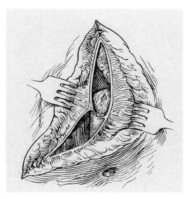

2. Incision continued through anterior rectus sheath, aponeurosis.

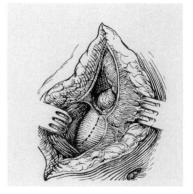

3. Exposure of posterior sheath. Incision follows dotted line.

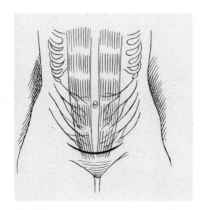

1. Pfannenstiel transverse elliptical incision used in gynecology.

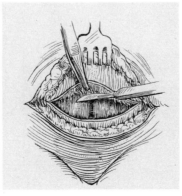

2. Anterior rectus sheath incised transversely, muscle separated.

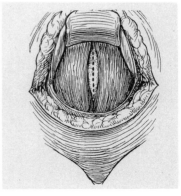

3. Posterior sheath and peritoneum are incised by vertical incision.

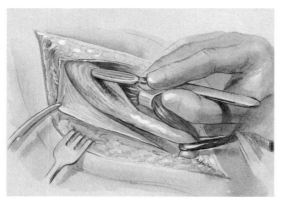

1. Aponeurosis of external oblique incised. Sac exposed by pushing back cremasteric fibres.

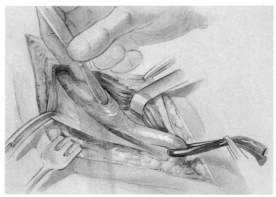

2. Internal spermatic fibres separated from internal ring by blunt dissection, exposing the hernial sac.

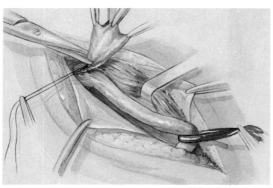

3. Hernial sac completely freed and ligature placed at its base. Sac now ready for removal.

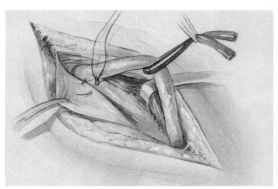

4. Transversalis fascia sutured to shelving edge of Poupart's. Note internal oblique muscle retracted.

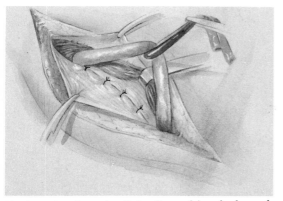

5. Completed repair of the floor of inguinal canal by means of fascia-to-fascia interrupted suture.

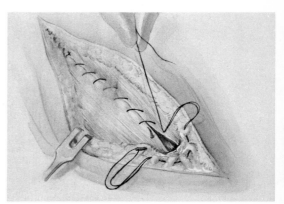

6. External oblique aponeurosis sutured. New external ring by purse-string suture in Scarpa's fascia.

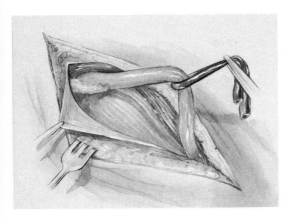

1. External oblique aponeurosis has been incised, exposing bulge in floor of inguinal canal.

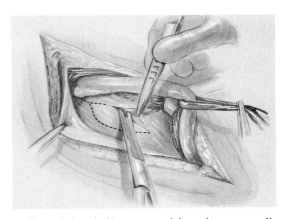

2. Dotted lines indicate area of frayed transversalis fibres over bulge to be excised, thus freeing hernia.

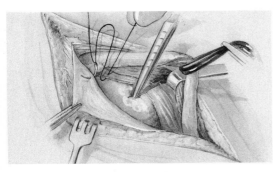

3. Transversalis fascia is sutured to shelving edge of Poupart's ligament as hernial sac is depressed.

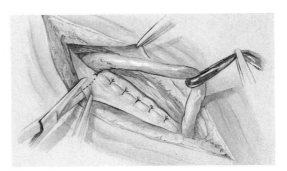

4. Flap for reinforcement of canal floor by transverse incision in lower flap of external oblique aponeurosis.

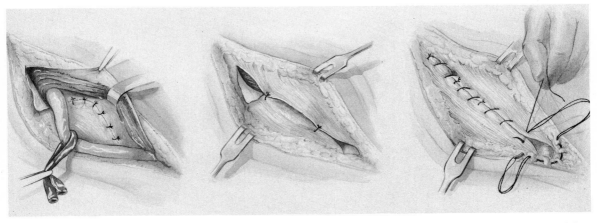

5. Fascial flap sutured over transversalis fascia.

6. Tension sutures hold upper flap of aponeurosis to external fold.

7. New external ring created by purse-string in Scarpa's fascia.

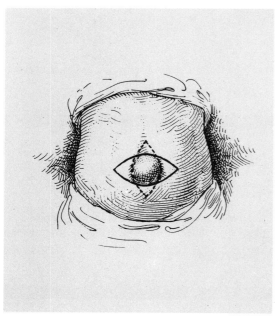

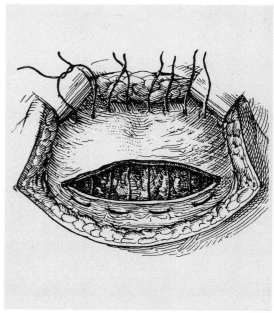

1. Surface anatomy and location and types of optional incisions indicated by solid and dotted lines.

2. Elliptic-transverse incision. Method of overlapping aponeurotic flap by multiple mattress sutures.

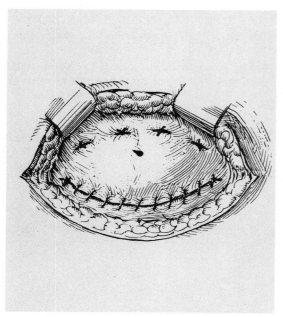

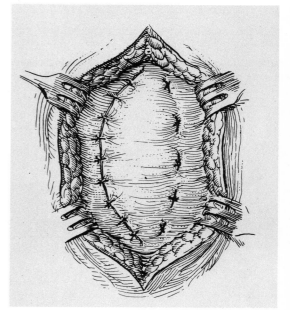

3. Mattress sutures completed and tied. The free edge of upper flap is secured by continuous suture.

4. Method of applying similar technique as described previously but utilizing elliptic-vertical incision.

REPAIR OF POSTOPERATIVE VENTRAL HERNIA
(JUDD)

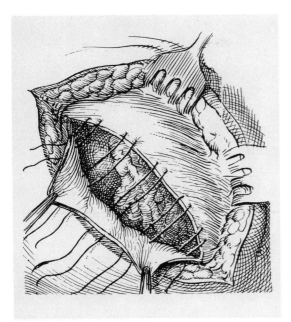

1. Incision completed. Aponeurosis freed, mattress sutures in place preparatory to overlapping of flap.

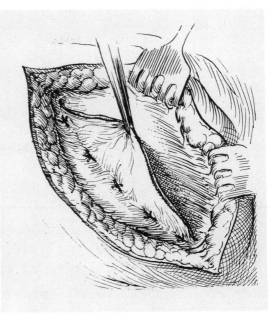

2. Mattress sutures have been completed. Extent of overlapping flap is demonstrated prior to suturing.

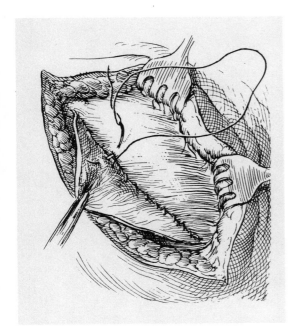

3. Reinforcement of mattress sutures by continuous suture placed on under surface of overlapping flap.

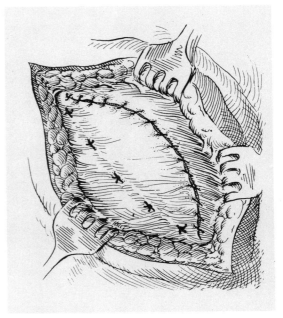

4. Aponeurosis sutures completed. Margin of flap sutured to aponeurosis by continuous technique.

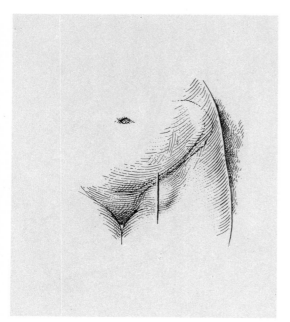

1. Surface anatomy and location of incision in relation to the femoral ring and the inguinal ligament.

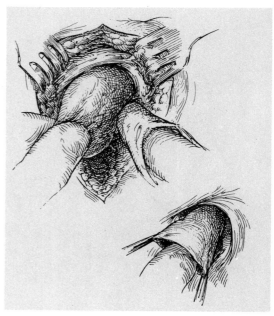

2. Sac isolated and freed by blunt dissection. Insert shows sac opened, contents in process of reduction.

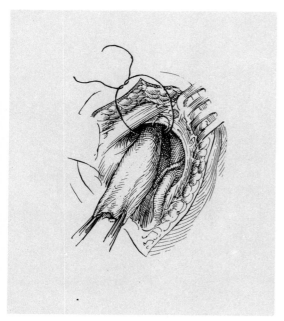

3. Reduction completed. Base of sac is ligated by means of transfixion suture prior to resection.

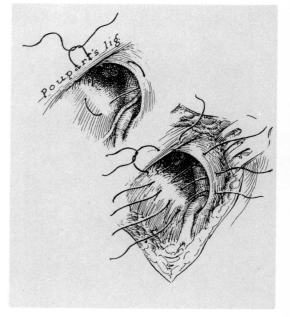

4. Closure. Purse-string or interrupted sutures approximate lacunar ligament to pectineus (Bassini).

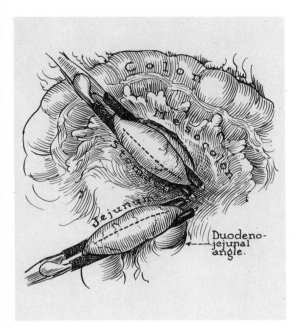

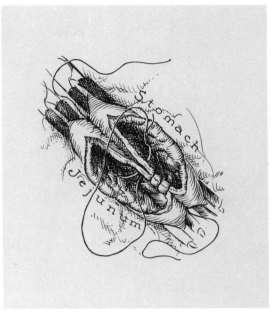

1. Rubber covered clamps applied to jejunum and stomach. Stomach drawn through slit in mesocolon.

2. Posterior seromuscular continuous suture completed. Posterior marginal suture is being placed.

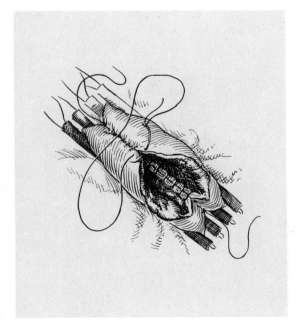

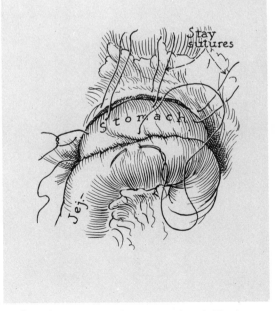

3. Anterior marginal suture is being placed. Note that long ends of seromuscular suture are preserved.

4. Anterior seromuscular suture placed. Tension sutures hold stomach in proper relation to mesocolon.

GASTROSTOMY
(STAMM METHOD)

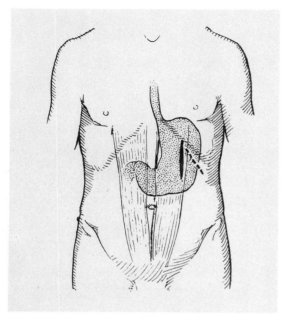

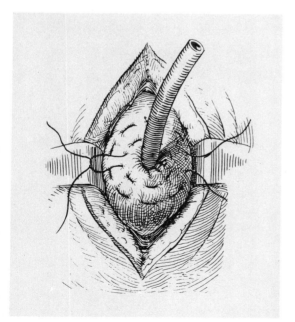

1. Location of skin incision and alternate incision in relation to left rectus muscle and stomach.

2. Method of introducing tube into stomach and fixing tube to stomach wall by means of single suture.

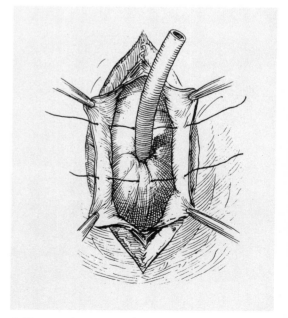

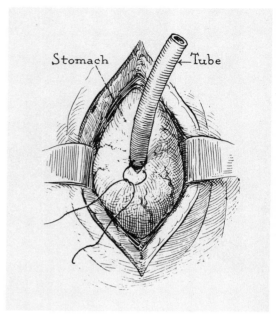

3. Method of placing three concentric rows of purse-string sutures in stomach wall around the tube.

4. Purse-string sutures tied beginning with proximal suture. Stomach fixed to anterior abdominal wall.

GASTROSTOMY
(DÉPAGE-JANEWAY)

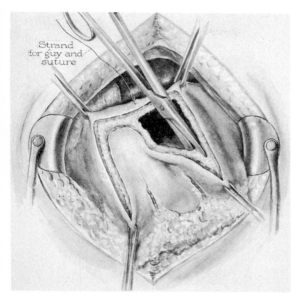

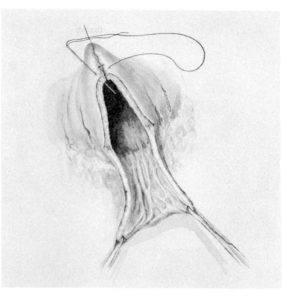

1. Allis forceps placed at angles of two-inch square. Serosa and muscularis have been incised.

2. Flap has been completed. Stomach approximated in transverse diameter by Connell sutures.

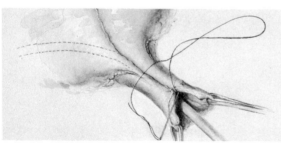

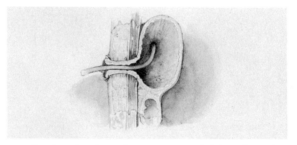

3. Suture continued transforming flap into tube. Rubber tube introduced extending into duodenum.

4. Section showing tube transplanted either through abdominal incision or left rectus stab wound.

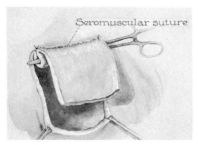

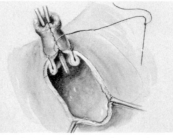

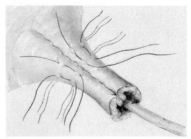

5. Alternative method after Spivack. Valve is formed at base.

6. Spivack method continued showing method of placing sutures.

7. Partipilo method of forming valve with Lembert sutures.

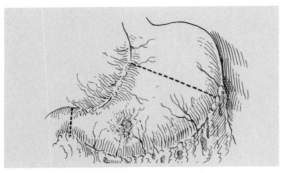

1. Diagram of stomach showing lesion. Dotted lines indicate section of stomach to be removed.

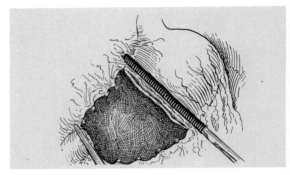

2. Portion of stomach has been clamped and resected. Duodenal stump is now prepared for inversion.

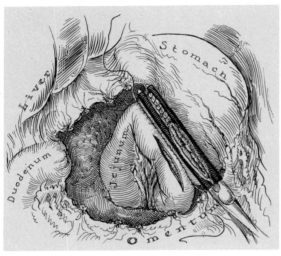

3. Duodenal invagination completed. Upper third of stomach closed. Jejunum brought through mesocolon.

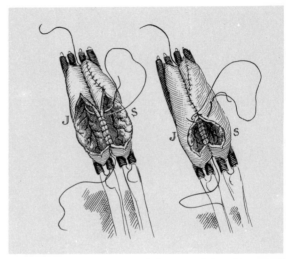

4. Establishing anastomosis between jejunal loop and lower two-thirds of incompleted stomach opening.

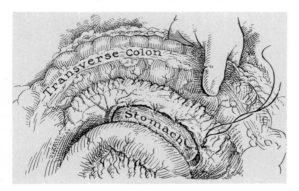

5. Gastro-jejuno anastomosis completed. The stomach is now fixed to the edges of slit in mesocolon.

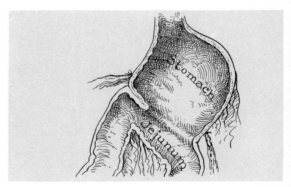

6. Cross section demonstrating completed operation showing anastomosis between stomach and jejunum.

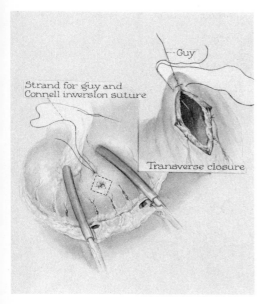

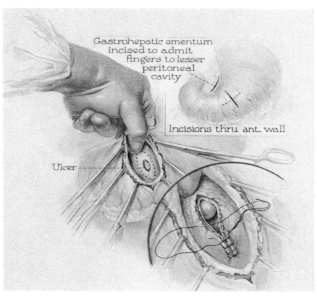

1. Diamond-shaped or square resection for ulcers on anterior wall indicated by dotted line.

2. Transgastric resection of ulcer on posterior wall. Posterior continuous lock suture: anterior inverting Connell.

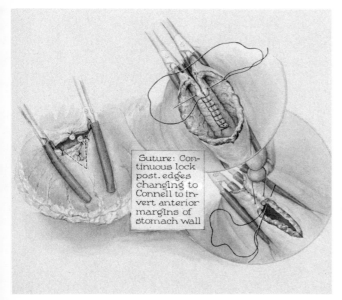

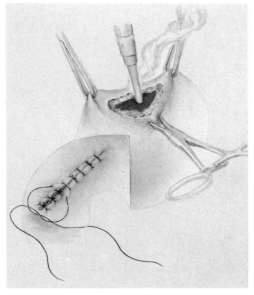

3. Dotted lines indicate wedge-shaped excision of ulcer on lesser curvature. The lesser omentum has been incised.

4. Cautery excision (Balfour). Closure by interrupted sutures, reinforced with mattress.

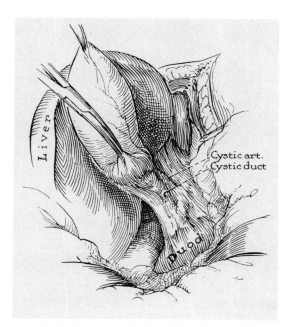

1. Gall bladder exposed, elevated by forceps. Second forceps exerts traction on pouch defining cystic duct.

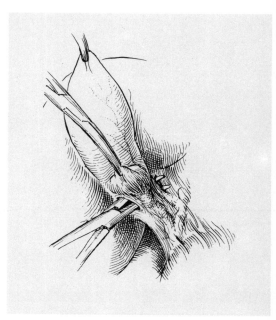

2. Cystic duct and artery isolated by passing forceps posterior to neck of gall bladder.

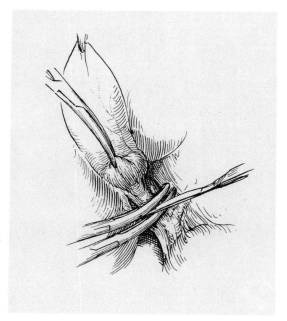

3. The cystic duct and artery are doubly clamped and ligated. Incision is made between the two clamps.

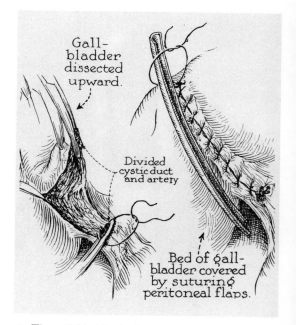

4. The gall bladder is dissected free from below upward. Closure of bladder bed, insertion of drain.

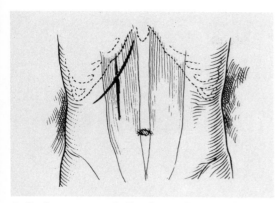

1. Surface anatomy indicating optional vertical and oblique incisions for exposure of gall bladder.

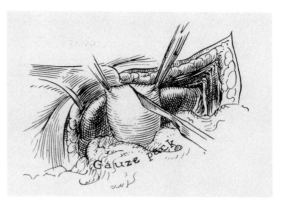

2. Gall bladder elevated, placed under tension. Gauze pack introduced, incision made into fundus.

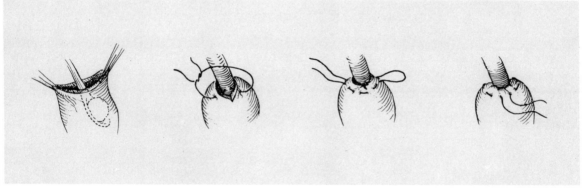

3. The fundus is opened and calculi removed. Drainage tube introduced and anchored by suture. Method of utilizing purse-string suture which does not include drainage tube.

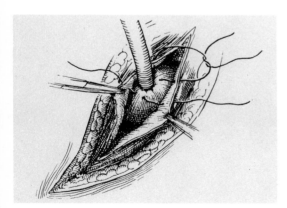

4. Anchoring fundus of gall bladder to peritoneum and fascia by means of interrupted sutures.

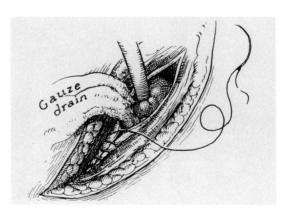

5. Alternate method of closure. Gall bladder is not anchored but dropped back into abdominal cavity.

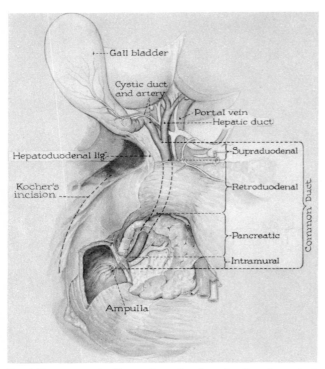

Semi-diagrammatic illustration showing details of surgical anatomy of extra-hepatic biliary tree. Kocher's incision.

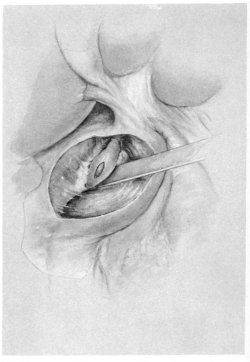

Incision exposing pancreatic and retroduodenal portion of common duct (Haasler).

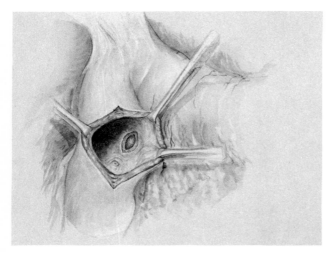

Kocher's transduodenal exposure completed. Pancreatic and intramural portions of duct visualized.

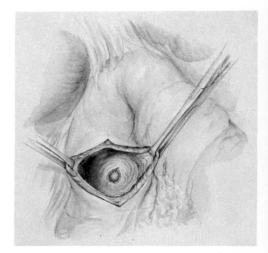

McBurney's transduodenal incision. Repair of meatus unnecessary. Drainage optional.

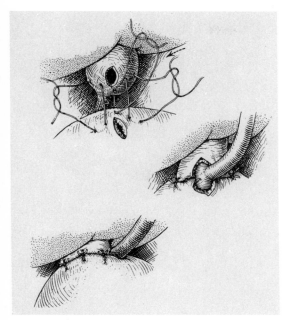

1. Direct anastomosis between dilated proximal portion of common duct and duodenum using "T" tube.

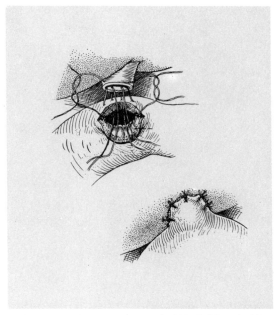

2. Modified direct anastomosis (W. J. Mayo). Flap from crescent in duodenum, sutured to liver capsule.

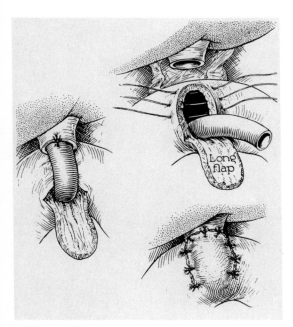

3. Progressive steps in cholecystoduodenostomy using rubber tube and long duodenal flap (Walton).

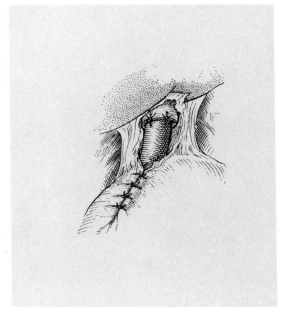

4. Jenckel method for cholecystoduodenostomy employing Witzel duodenostomy.

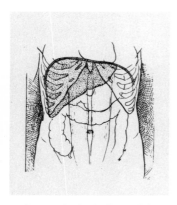

1. Anatomical relations of liver to ribs and adjacent structures.

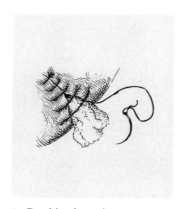

2. Combined continuous suture and gauze tampon.

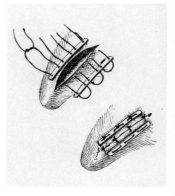

3. Marginal wound closure using magnesium plates.

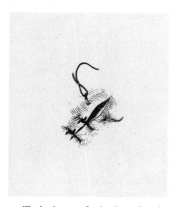

4. Technique of placing simple interrupted sutures.

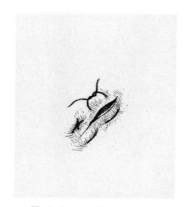

5. Technique of placing mattress sutures.

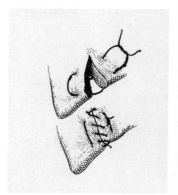

6. Suture of liver margin reinforced by continuous suture.

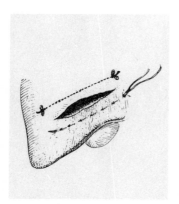

7. Parallel sunken strands as traction sutures along defect.

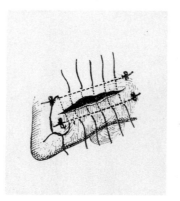

8. Placing interrupted sutures transversely to sunken strands.

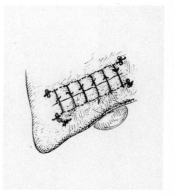

9. Relationship of transverse sutures to sunken strands.

SPLENECTOMY

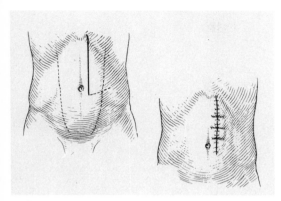

1. Paramedian incision with Kocher extension. Closure without drainage using tension sutures.

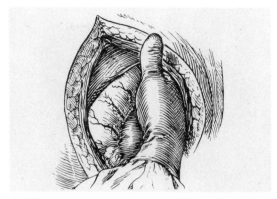

2. Right hand inserted to mobilize spleen from phrenic and posterior attachments.

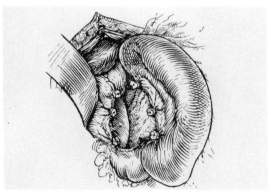

3. Vasa brevia ligated and gastrosplenic ligament divided, aiding mobilization and exposing pedicle.

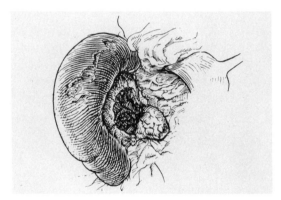

4. Spleen reflected mesially. Tail of pancreas freed from pedicle, exposing main splenic vessels.

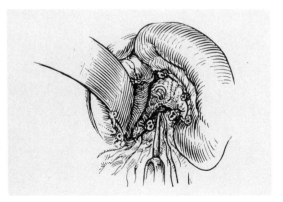

5. Vessels of pedicle serially ligated. Procedure often facilitated by use of ligature carrier.

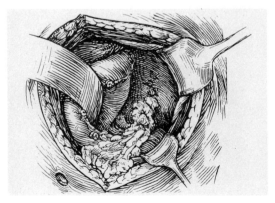

6. Omental fat sutured to stump of pedicle insuring hemostasis and obliterating dead space.

END TO END ENTERO-ENTEROSTOMY
(CLOSED METHOD OF PARKER-KERR)

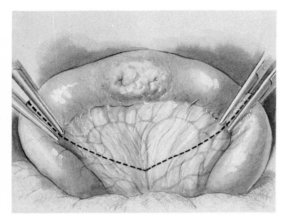

1. Site of lesion and placing of two sets of clamps. Dotted lines indicate area for excision.

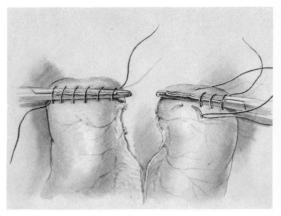

2. Method of placing continuous inverting suture over clamps. Ends of suture are left long.

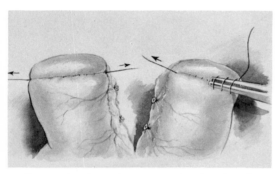

3. Completing inverting sutures by drawing them taut as opened clamp is gradually withdrawn.

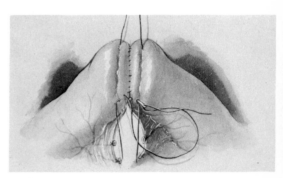

4. Inversion completed. Continuous serosal suture placed and the musculo-serous stitch begun.

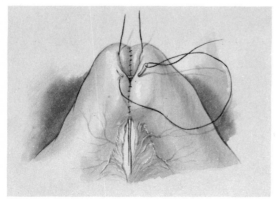

5. Posterior musculo-serous suture placed. This suture now continued to approximate anterior surface.

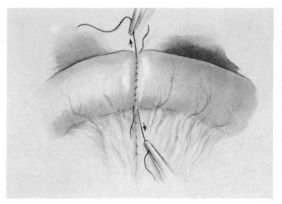

6. Serous suture completed, mesentery approximated. Original inverting sutures are now withdrawn.

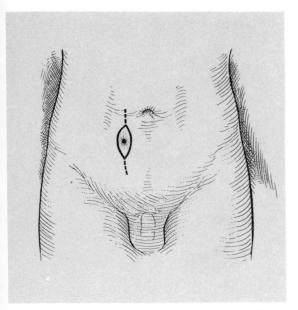

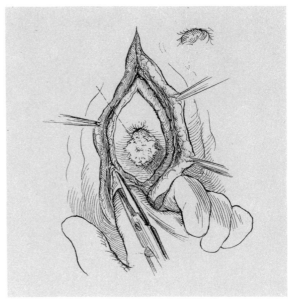

1. Surface anatomy demonstrating elliptical incision surrounding opening of fistulous tract.

2. Collodian covered gauze plug in fistula. Finger explores relations as excision of tract is completed.

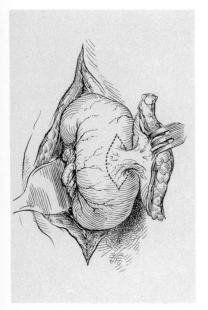

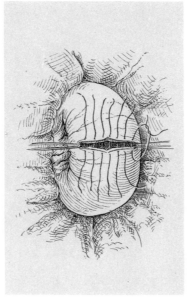

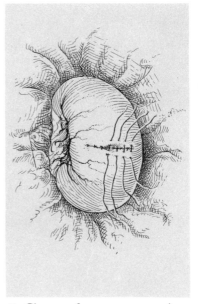

3. Neck of tract exposed, separated from intestine along dotted line.

4. Longitudinal converted into transverse opening for patency.

5. Closure of transverse opening with interrupted inverting sutures.

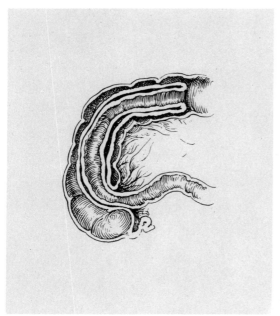

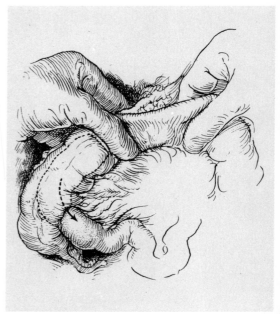

1. Diagrammatic sagittal section showing mechanics of intussusception. Invagination of the ileum into colon.

2. Reduction by firm but gentle pressure on head of invaginated portion, correcting invagination.

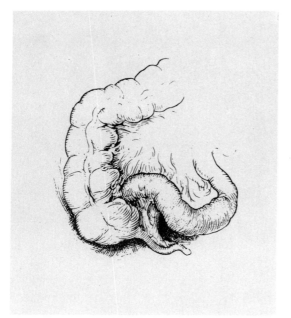

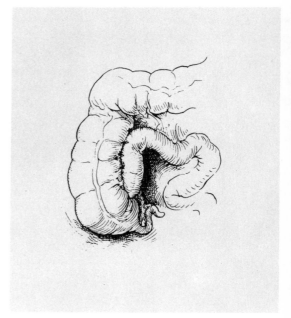

3. Reduction completed. Intestine found to be viable, and resection of ileum therefore unnecessary.

4. Optional method of suturing portion of ileum to ascending colon as means of preventing recurrence.

ARTIFICIAL ANUS WITH SUBTOTAL COLECTOMY
(SPIVACK)

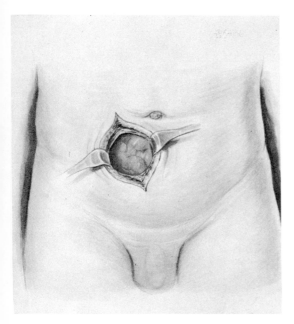

1. Surface anatomy showing right pararectus incision for exposure of the ileocecal region.

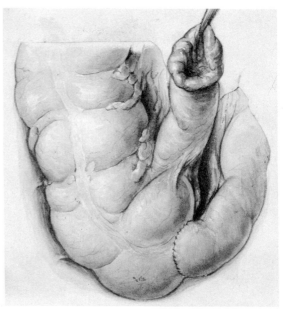

2. Terminal ileum divided eight centimeters from ileocecal valve and proximal end implanted into cecum.

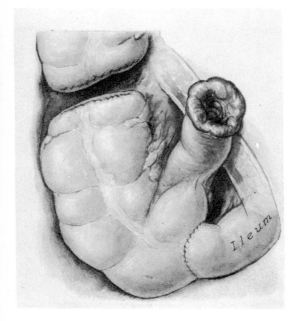

3. Distal end of ileum brought through abdominal wall. Colon divided preparatory to subtotal colectomy.

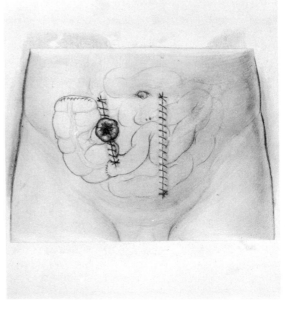

4. Artificial anus and closure of left paramedian incision through which colectomy was performed.

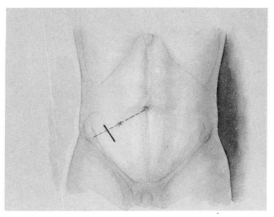

1. Location of McBurney incision in relation to line between anterior superior spine and the umbilicus.

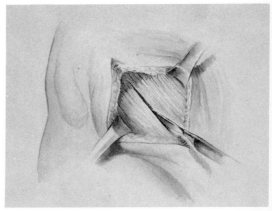

2. Line of incision of external oblique aponeurosis which is in same direction as the fibres.

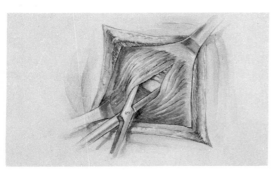

3. Direction of incision is now changed to follow fibres of internal oblique and transversalis muscles.

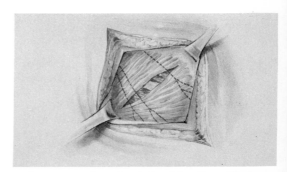

4. Demonstration of relationship of twelfth intercostal nerve to the line of incision.

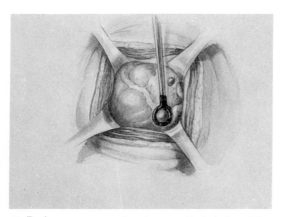

5. Peritoneum opened and appendix is being delivered by rubber covered forceps at base of cecum.

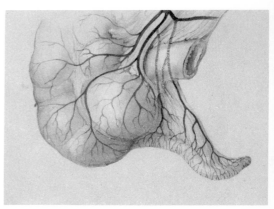

6. Anatomy of the ileocecal region showing relationship of meso-appendix and appendiceal arteries.

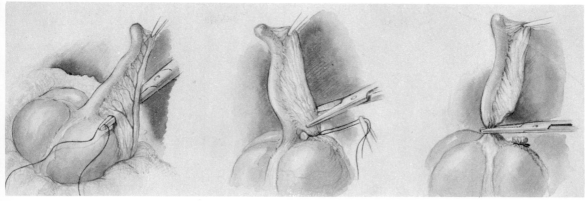

1. Cecum walled off. Ligature passed through meso-appendix.

2. Meso-appendix ligated, cut. Multiple clamps may be used.

3. Meso-appendix separated. Clamp placed at base of appendix.

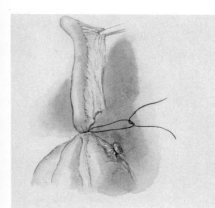

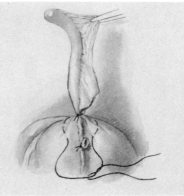

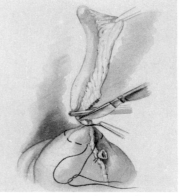

4. Crushing clamp removed and groove left in base is now ligated.

5. Purse-string suture at base. Appendix ready for amputation.

6. Clamp distal to ligature. Appendix amputated with carbolic knife.

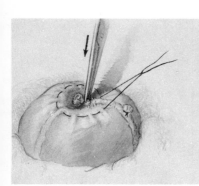

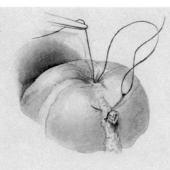

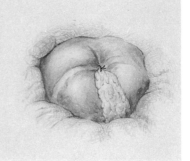

7. Appendiceal stump inverted as purse-string suture is tied.

8. Suture of ileocecal fat pad or mesentery to protect stump.

9. Operation completed. Alternate method omits purse-string suture.

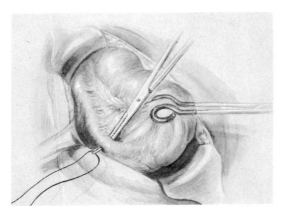

1. Cecum delivered into wound and rotated mesially. Ligature drawn under base of appendix.

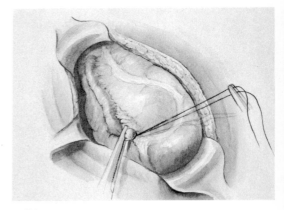

2. Ligature tied and ends left long. Crushing clamp placed on appendix slightly distal to ligature.

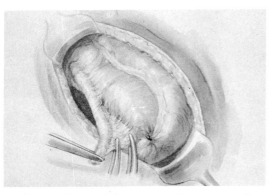

3. Stump inverted by purse-string suture. Removal of appendix by multiple clamp method.

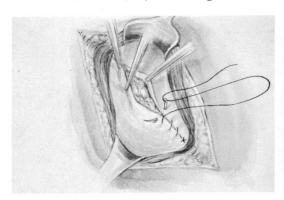

4. Omentum is drawn over the cecum. Peritoneum is closed by means of continuous suture.

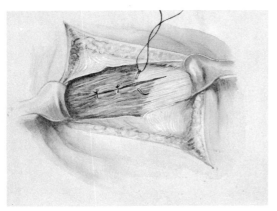

5. Loose interrupted sutures are used to approximate the internal oblique and transversalis muscles.

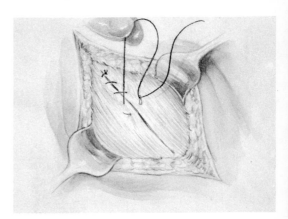

6. Closure of external oblique aponeurosis by either continuous or continuous interrupted technique.

PARTIAL RESECTION OF COLON
(MIKULICZ)

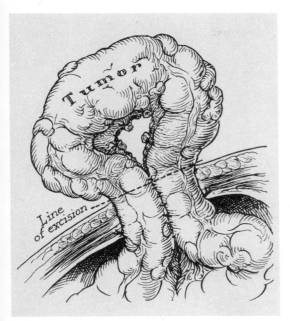

1. Loop of bowel to be resected delivered through wound. Note suture to form spur.

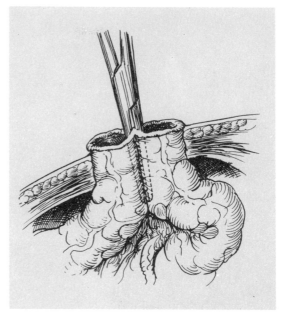

2. Method of gradual application of crushing clamp to spur five to nine days after resection has been done.

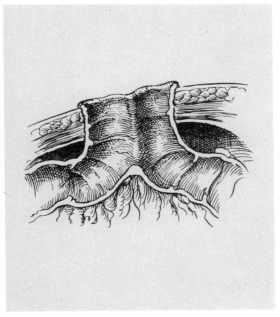

3. Cross-sectional view demonstrating spur broken down. The bowel is now ready for permanent closure.

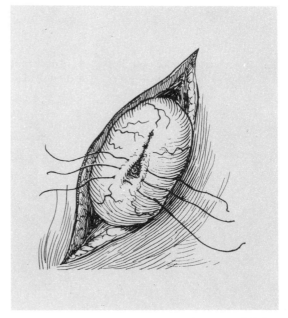

4. Bowel freed extraperitoneally. Closure of defect effected by interrupted inverting sutures.

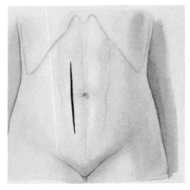

1. Surface anatomy and extent of right paramedian incision.

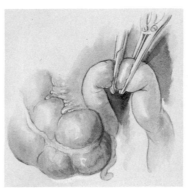

2. Ileocecal region showing clamp placed on distal portion of ileum.

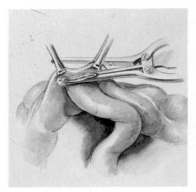

3. Ileum brought to position for anastomosis to transverse colon.

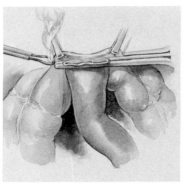

4. Rankin clamp in position. Portion of taenia removed by cautery.

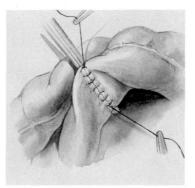

5. Anastomosis begun. Posterior sero-muscular suture. Ends long.

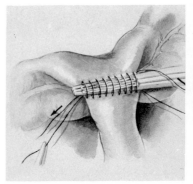

6. Inverting suture over clamps. Long sutures to be removed.

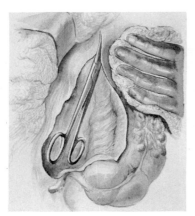

7. Mobilization of right colon by incising of peritoneal reflection.

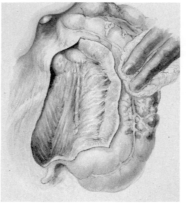

8. Continued dissection of colon exposing right kidney and ureter.

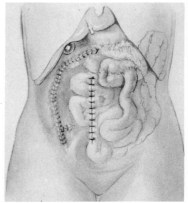

9. Completed anastomosis. Note closure of lateral peritoneal gutter.

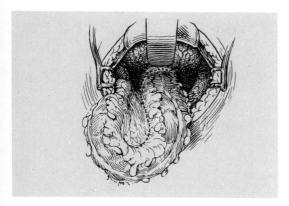

1. Initial step in abdomino-perineal resection of rectum. Dotted line indicates incision in peritoneum.

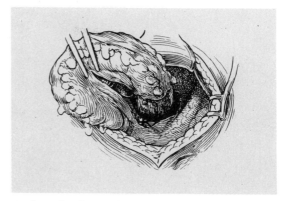

2. Superior hemorrhoidal artery ligated and cut. Bowel clamped preparatory to division.

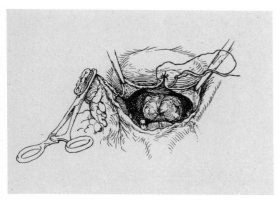

3. Distal end of bowel has been closed and deposited in pelvis, and the peritoneum closed over it.

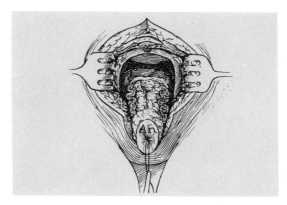

4. Perineal dissection. Coccyx excised. Levator ani muscles divided, and pelvic fascia opened.

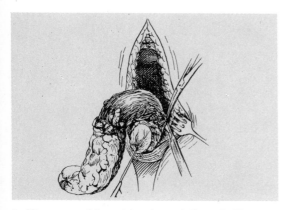

5. The resected bowel has been delivered. The anal end of the rectum is freed by sharp dissection.

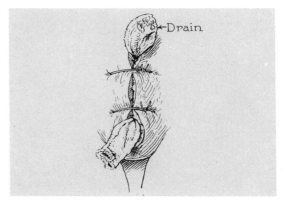

6. Method of closing perineal wound by gauze pack covered with oiled silk. Use of sutures optional.

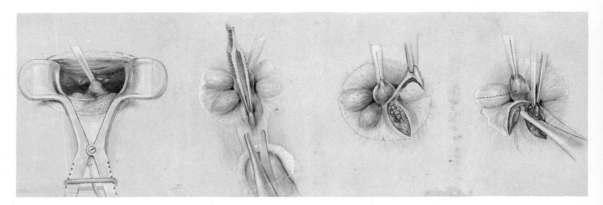

1. Dilator in place and internal hemorrhoid grasped with forceps. Skin over external hemorrhoid elevated with tissue forceps. Redundant skin is cut up to the mucocutaneous line. Veins are dissected from hemorrhoid.

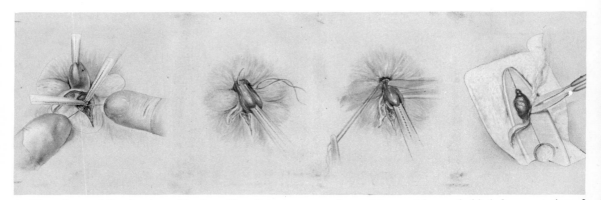

2. Clamping and ligating large bleeders. Transfixion suture at base of internal hemorrhoid tied, amputation of hemorrhoid distal to ligation. Alternate method using hemorrhoid clamp and cautery shown at right.

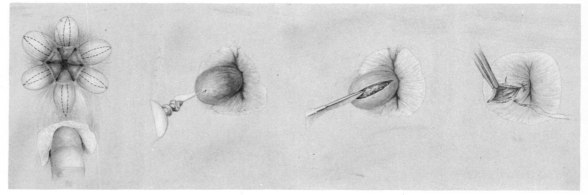

3. Scheme of skin excision following radiating lines. Enucleation of thrombosed external hemorrhoid. Injection of local anesthetic. Incision for removal of thrombus. Closure of skin by interrupted sutures optional.

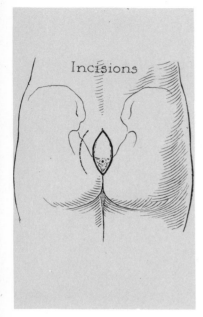

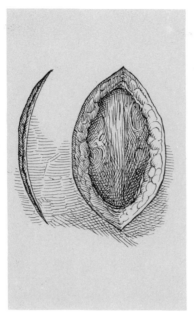

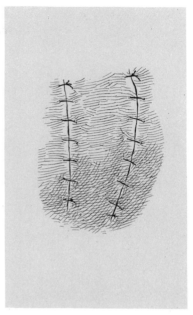

1. Dye injected into sinuses. Accessory incision shown (Lahey).

2. Wide excision completed. Wound packed. Sutures optional.

3. Bridge of skin and fat displaced to midline. Lateral defect sutured.

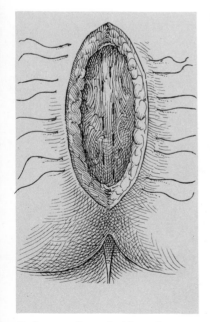

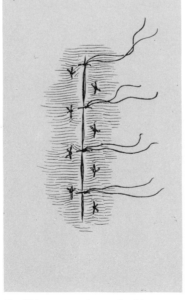

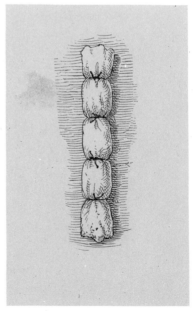

1. Sutures through skin and sacro-coccygeal ligaments (Colp).

2. Skin approximated. Alternate method omits use of sutures.

3. Pressure dressing tied in place by long ends of sutures.

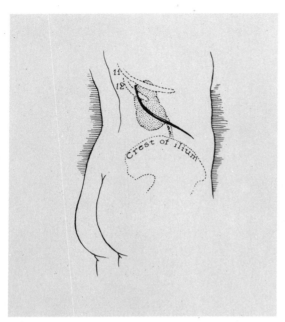

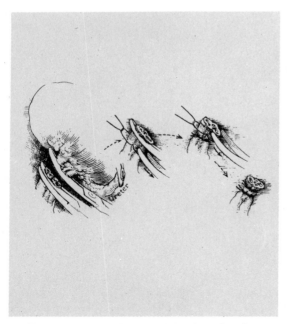

1. Surface anatomy, kidney outlined. Location of incision in relation to twelfth rib and crest of ileum.

2. Horizontal cross section at level of incision showing relations of kidney to surrounding structures.

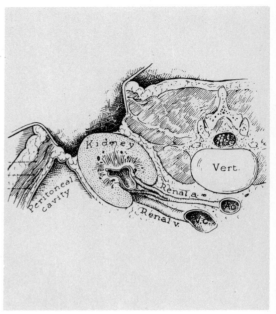

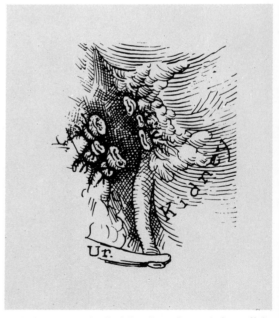

3. Serial steps in clamping and ligation of pedicle en masse by means of figure of eight transfixion suture.

4. Alternate method of ligation of vessels in pedicle by means of separate ligature for each vessel.

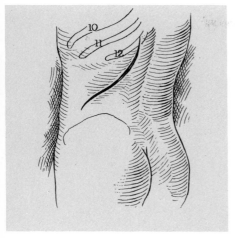

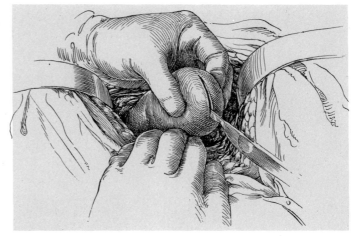

1. Location of skin incision for wide exposure and relationship to 12th rib.

2. Incision completed and wound margins retracted. Kidney is now immobilized. Nephrotomy incision made in lower pole.

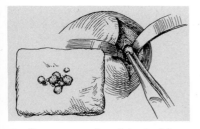

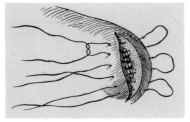

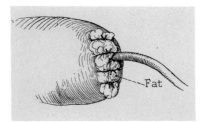

3. Retractors placed in incision. Stones removed by tissue forceps.

4. Kidney incision is closed in two layers. Mattress sutures in place.

5. Alternate method of kidney closure using fat pad and drainage.

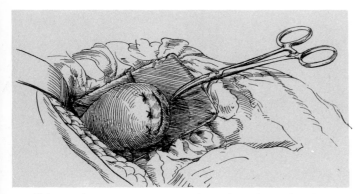

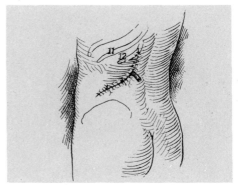

6. Prior to closure, roentgenogram is made to determine that all stones have been removed. Sterile film holder in place.

7. Closure showing interrupted skin sutures and drainage of perinephric space.

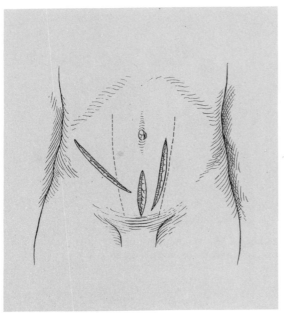

1. Types of incision commonly used for gaining access to lower portion of ureter and to bladder.

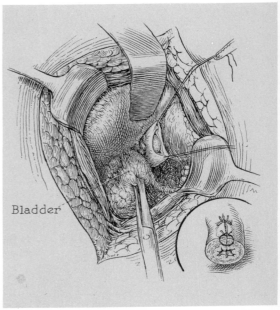

2. Extra-peritoneal removal of ureteral stone. Cross section of ureter and method of placing sutures.

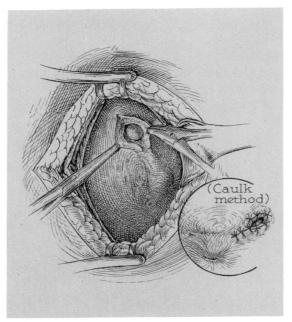

3. Intravesical removal of intramural stone through low midline incision. Method of suturing bladder.

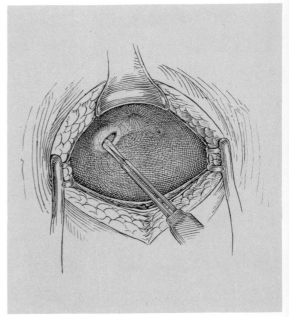

4. Low midline incision. Intravesical stone removed by cautery method. No sutures used.

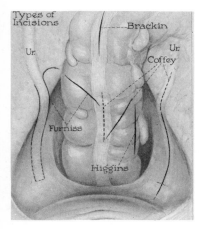

1. Location of incision and optional incisions commonly employed.

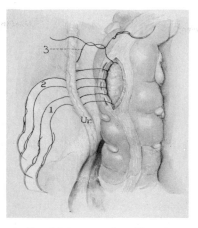

2. Brackin's operation. First 3 sutures by double needle technique.

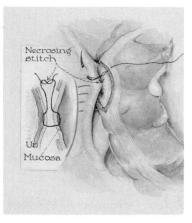

3. Second step. Necrosing stitch between ureter and colon mucosa.

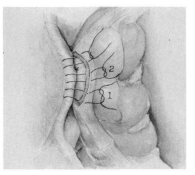

4. Demonstration of non-constricting feature of mattress sutures.

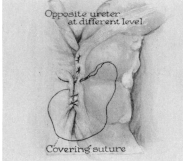

5. Continuous covering suture. Continuity of ureter is maintained.

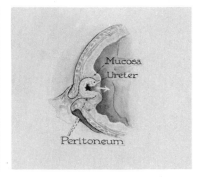

6. Cross section. Final result after necrosing stitch has sloughed.

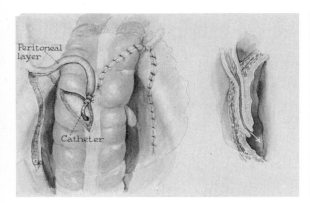

Uretero-intestinal anastamosis. Following Furniss' modification of Coffey's technique. Note catheter.

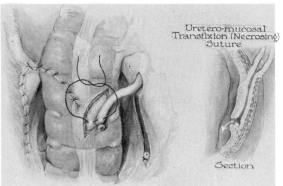

Alternate method. Placement of necrosing suture is illustrated. Continuity of ureter is interrupted.

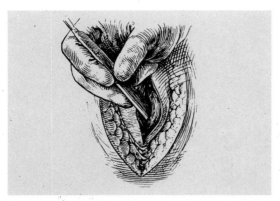

1. Low suprapubic incision carried through fascia. The recti muscles separated by blunt dissection.

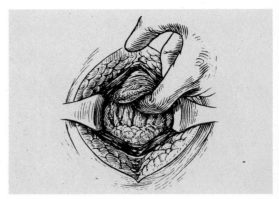

2. The muscles and fascia are retracted laterally, and the peritoneal fold is separated from the bladder.

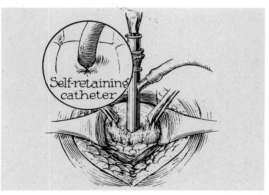

3. Bladder supported by Allis clamps. Method of insertion of trocar for cystostomy drainage.

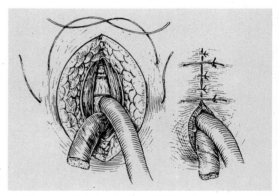

4. Closure of abdominal wall following cystostomy in one or two layers. Note prevesical drain.

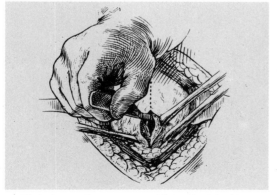

5. Technique of cystotomy. Abdominal incision as above. The bladder is incised from below upward.

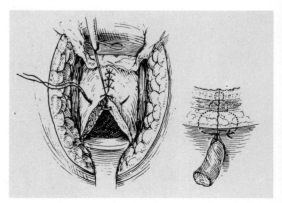

6. Suture of bladder by interrupted technique. Three-layer abdominal closure and prevesical drain.

CIRCUMCISION

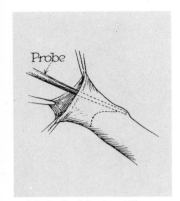

1. Method of freeing adherent prepuce from glans.

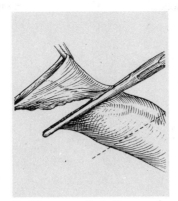

2. Clamp applied. Prepuce incised parallel with corona.

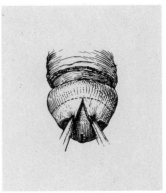

3. Outer layer retracted, inner trimmed along dotted line.

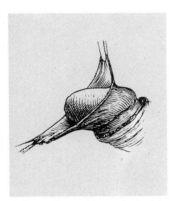

4. Inner layer trimmed to within one centimeter of corona.

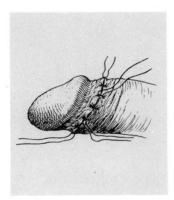

5. Method of suturing. Alternate sutures left long.

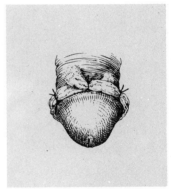

6. Long ends of suture used to hold vaseline gauze dressing.

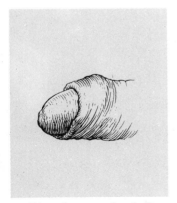

7. Operation completed. Prepuce partially covers the glans.

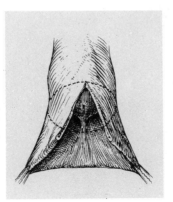

8. Alternate method of circumcision utilizing dorsal slit.

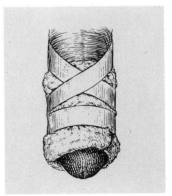

9. Closure by continuous suture. Vaseline gauze dressing.

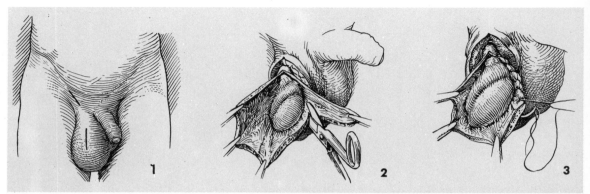

1. Surface anatomy and location of optional incisions. **2.** Method of trimming redundant tunica. **3.** Technique of placing continuous hemostatic suture in margin of remaining tunica.

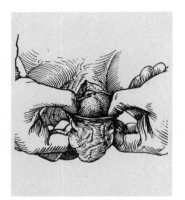
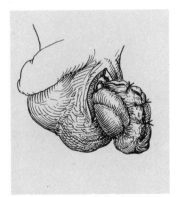
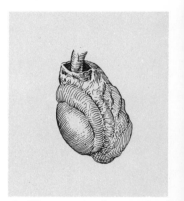

4. Alternate method. Testicle pushed through opening in sac.

5. Alternate method. Tunica turned inside out and sutured.

6. Diagram showing result of everting sac upon cord.

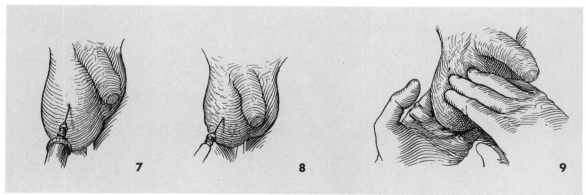

7. First step in injection method. Aspiration of fluid by means of syringe. **8.** Fluid has been removed and sclerosing solution is being injected. **9.** Gentle massage of scrotum to facilitate action of sclerosing solution.

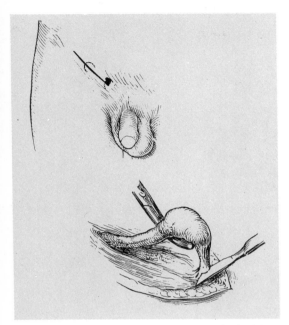

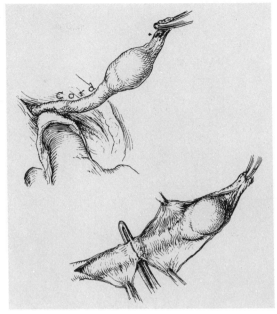

1. Surface anatomy and location of skin incision. Cord and testicle freed. Gubernaculum severed.

2. Cord freed by blunt dissection. Grooved director introduced between tunica vaginalis and cord.

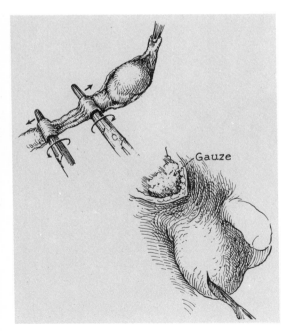

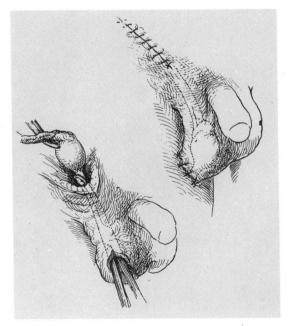

3. Method of stripping tunica vaginalis from cord using clamps. Incision of scrotal sac.

4. Gubernaculum grasped and pulled into scrotum through incision and anchored to fascia of thigh.

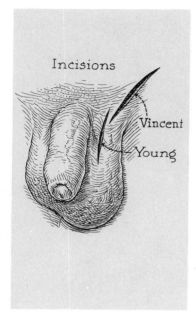

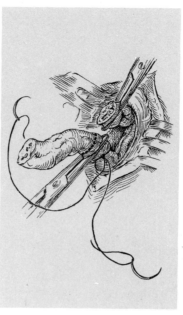

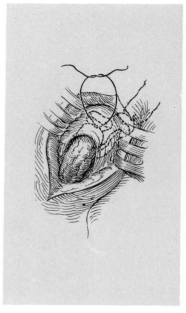

1. Location and types of optional incisions commonly used.

2. Vincent technique: preservation of vas, artery, and one vein.

3. Proximal stump dropped back, distal suspended to external ring.

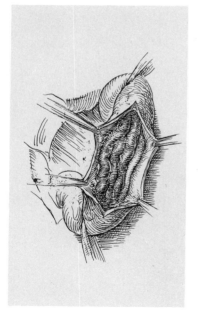

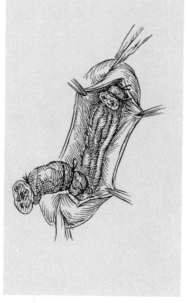

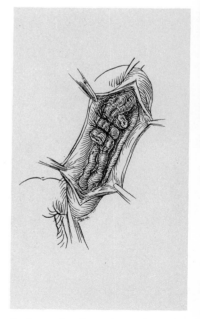

1. Young's technique. Cord is drawn upward. Dartos is opened.

2. Redundant veins dissected, doubly ligated, prepared for excision.

3. Severed vein ends are brought together, overlapped and sutured.

ABDOMINAL HYSTERECTOMY
(CURTIS)

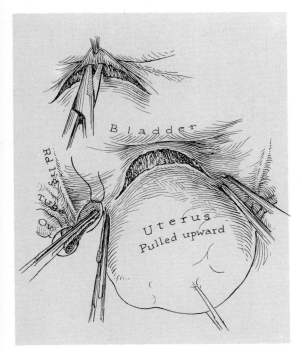

1. Prevesical peritoneum incised and dissected. Double clamping of tubes and round ligaments.

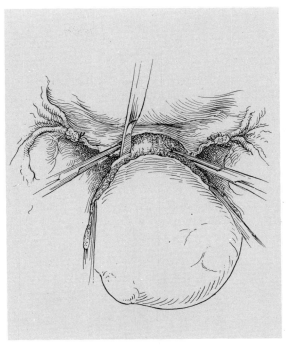

2. Broad ligaments ligated by figure of eight stitch. Uterine arteries clamped, including bite into cervix.

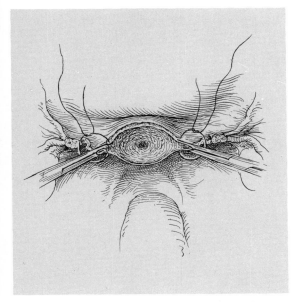

3. Uterine arteries ligated by sutures, including portion of cervical stump. Amputation conical incision.

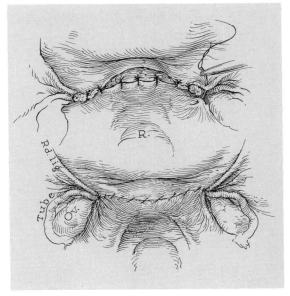

4. Incision margins approximated by interrupted sutures. Peritonealization of entire area completed.

VAGINAL HYSTERECTOMY
(DÖDERLEIN-KRÖNIG-GRAVES)

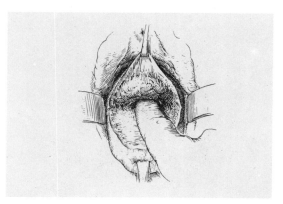

1. Transverse incision at cysto-cervical junction. Bladder is pushed back by finger.

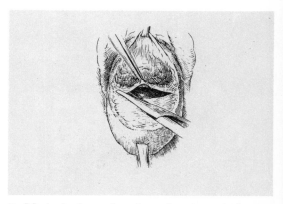

2. Method of opening through uterovesical space using scissors. Note bladder above.

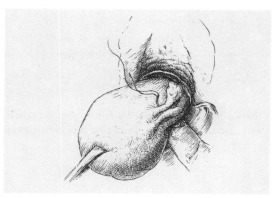

3. Fundus grasped and delivered through incision. Adnexa ligated with mass transfixion ligatures.

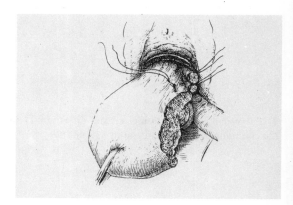

4. Broad ligament divided close to uterus. Uterine artery ligated. Transfixion ligatures left long.

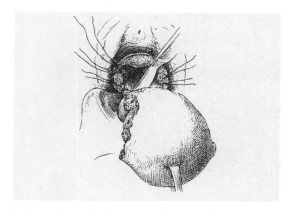

5. Anterior vaginal wall has been divided. Parametrium and posterior vaginal wall being incised.

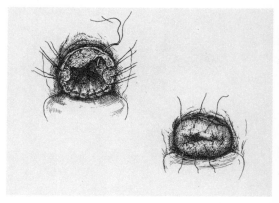

6. Broad ligaments sutured to vaginal wall. Peritonealization and method of closure of vagina.

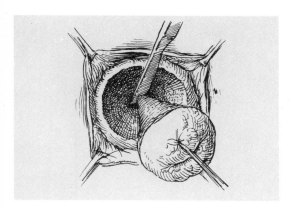

1. Sturmdorf method. Tenaculum applied and conical excision made up to level of the internal os.

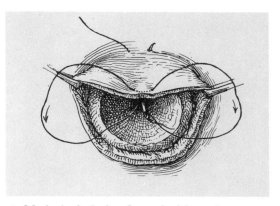

2. Method of placing Sturmdorf inverting suture. Sufficient mucosa is allowed to cover raw surface.

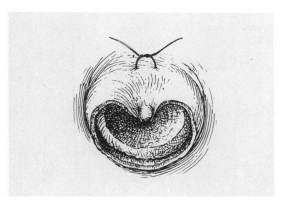

3. First Sturmdorf inverting suture. Similar posterior and lateral sutures to be placed.

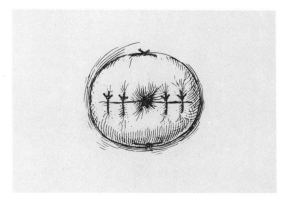

4. Inverting mucosal sutures completed. Mucosa is approximated by additional interrupted sutures.

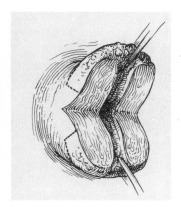

5. Curtis-Schroeder method. Cervix is incised horizontally.

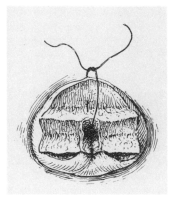

6. Portion removed above and below the horizontal split.

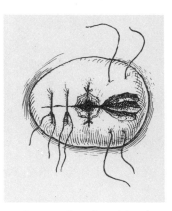

7. Raw surface closed by deep and mucosal sutures.

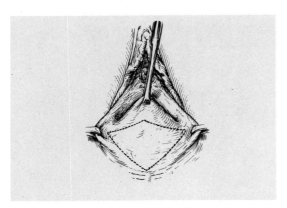

1. Clamps placed laterally below Bartholin glands. Dotted line indicates Hegar's pattern of excision.

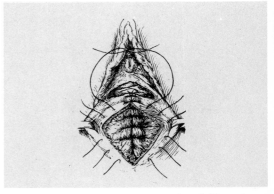

2. Hegar closure. Excision completed. Deep interrupted sutures approximate levator muscles.

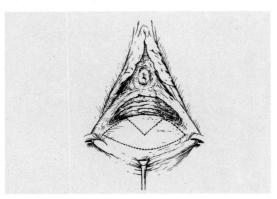

1. Emmet-Studdiford method. Allis clamps placed laterally and posterially at mucocutaneous junction.

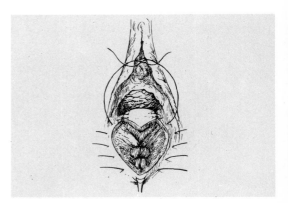

2. Interrupted sutures approximating levator ani muscles. Interrupted mucosal sutures at apex.

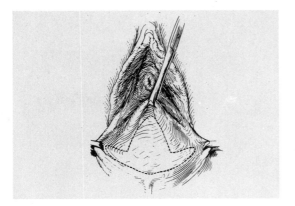

1. Clark method. Allis clamps in place. Dotted line indicates pattern of mucosal excision.

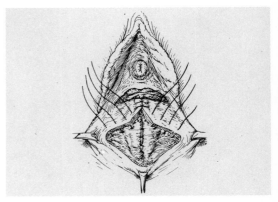

2. Interrupted levator sutures completed. Mucosal closure by interrupted sutures in vertical line.

MEDIAN EPISIOTOMY AND REPAIR
(MATSNER)

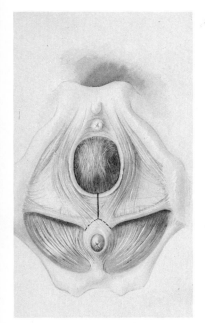

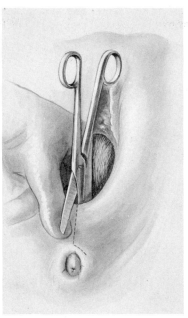

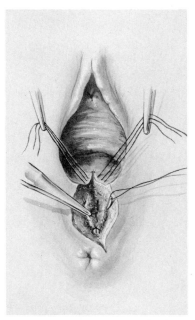

1. Midline incision. Dotted lines indicate optional extensions.

2. Incision made with bandage scissors to avoid fetal trauma.

3. Mucosal sutures placed. Approximation of levator muscles.

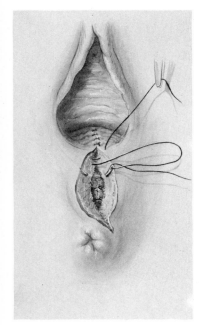

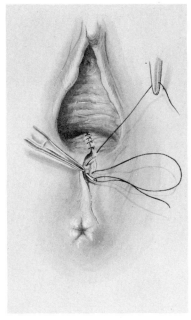

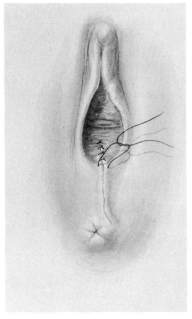

4. Long subcutaneous suture inserted at mucocutaneous line.

5. Same suture is utilized for skin closure by subcuticular stitch.

6. Subcuticular suture completed and tied at mucocutaneous line.

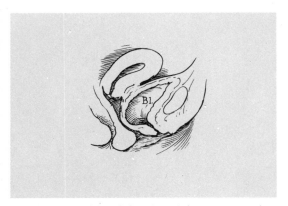

1. Sagittal section of female pelvis demonstrating presence of cystocele.

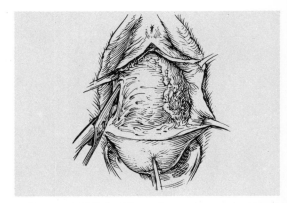

2. Inverted "T" incision of anterior vaginal wall and cervix. Bladder pillars separated.

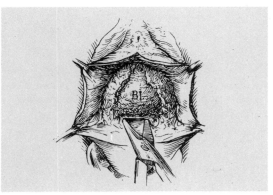

3. Bladder pillars and parametrium separated from vaginal flaps. The bladder is freed by blunt dissection.

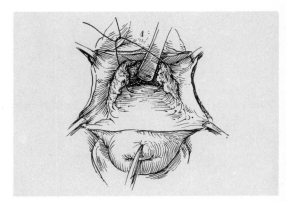

4. Bladder elevated. Bladder pillars and parametrium united. Sutures include bite into uterus.

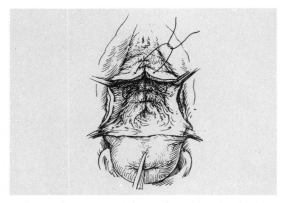

5. Redundant mucosal flaps trimmed and united by interrupted sutures which include underlying tissue.

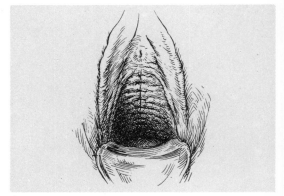

6. The operation completed showing suture line in anterior vaginal wall and obliteration of cystocele.

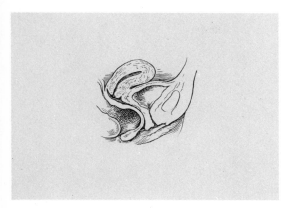

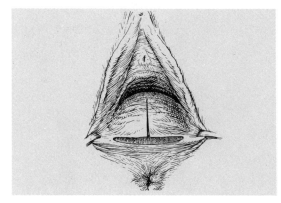

1. Sagittal cross section of female pelvis showing anatomy and presence of second degree rectocele.

2. Vertical incision of vaginal mucosa. Small strip of mucocutaneous junction removed horizontally.

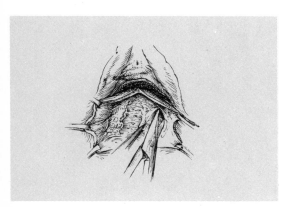

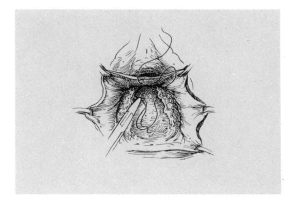

3. Allis clamps placed on mucous membrane. Rectovaginal fascia dissected bluntly from vaginal mucosa.

4. Purse-string suture at apex includes vaginal mucosa as well as the rectovaginal fascia.

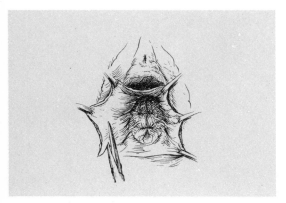

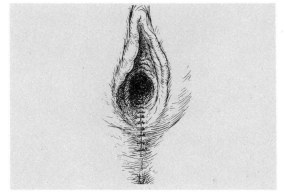

5. The rectocele has been obliterated by a series of sutures. The redundant mucosal flaps are trimmed.

6. Operation completed. Row of interrupted sutures in vertical line approximates both mucosa and skin.

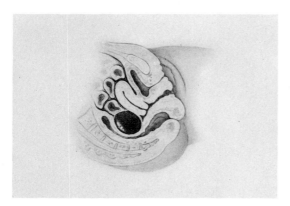

1. Sagittal section demonstrating intraperitoneal type of pelvic abscess in pouch of Douglas.

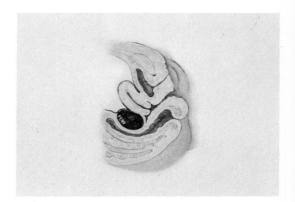

2. Sagittal section demonstrating extraperitoneal type of pelvic abscess in pouch of Douglas.

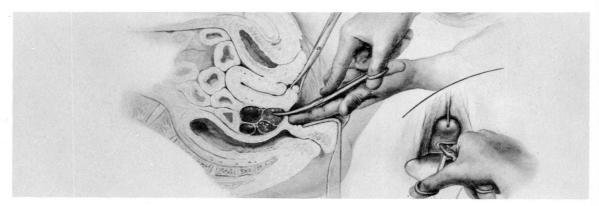

3. Posterior fornix made tense by traction on posterior lip of cervix. Sharp curved scissors are used to penetrate the vaginal wall. Following penetration, scissor blades are separated to extend opening.

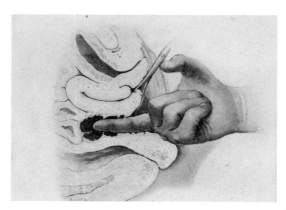

4. Method of using finger introduced into abscess cavity to break up loculations.

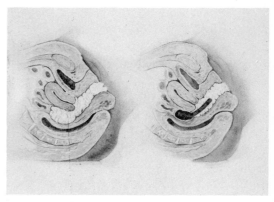

5. Two methods of drainage. Gauze pack of cavity and vagina. Tube in cavity and vagina packed.

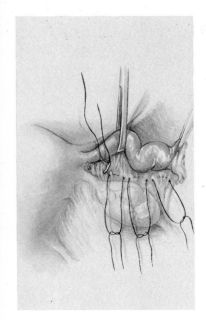

1. Method of placing transfixion sutures in broad ligament.

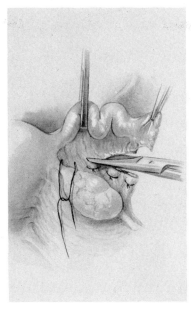

2. Transfixion sutures tied. Broad ligament incised with scissors.

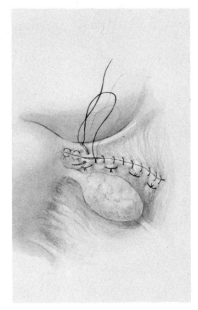

3. Method of peritonealizing tubal stump and broad ligament.

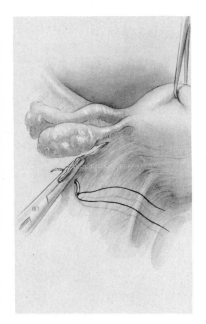

4. First step in salpingo-oophorectomy. Transfixion sutures placed.

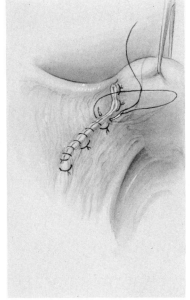

5. Covering raw surface of broad ligament, peritonealization.

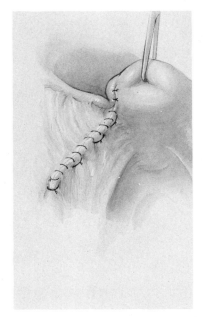

6. Completed operation. Round ligament sutured over stump.

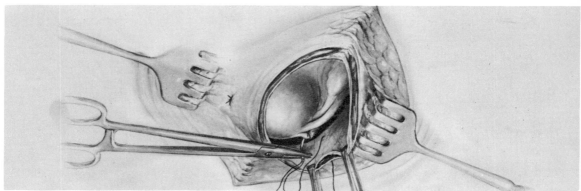

1. Approach by low midline or Pfannenstiel incision. Suture is placed under proximal end of round ligament and brought through all layers of anterior abdominal wall up to subcutaneous tissue (Olshausen).

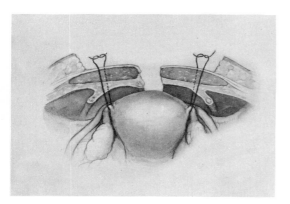

2. Cross section diagram showing suspension completed as described above (Kelly's modification).

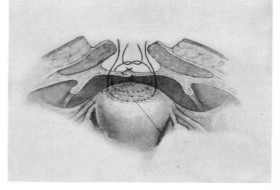

3. Sutures pass through fundus attaching it to peritoneum and posterior rectus sheath (Leopold).

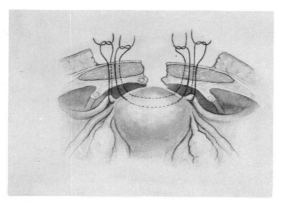

4. Uterus fixed by round ligament and fundus sutures through anterior rectus sheath (Vineberg).

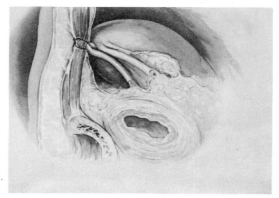

5. Sagittal section demonstrating completed operation and uterine fixation to anterior abdominal wall.

OPERATION FOR RECURRENT DISLOCATION
OF SHOULDER
(NICOLA)

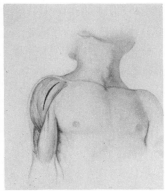

1. Anatomy showing incision in relation to underlying muscle.

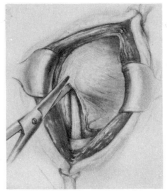

2. Exposure of tendon of long head of the biceps.

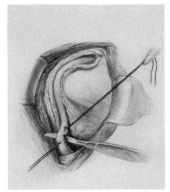

3. Tension sutures placed. Tendon cut below bicipital groove.

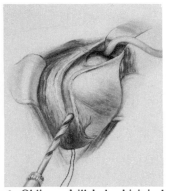

4. Oblique drill hole; bicipital groove to anatomical neck.

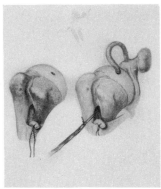

5. Method of threading proximal tendon end through hole.

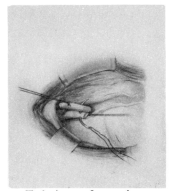

6. Technique of suturing cut ends of tendon with overlap.

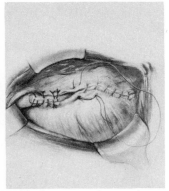

7. Tendon sutured to periosteum. Bicipital groove closed.

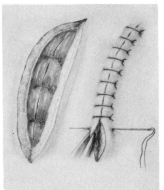

8. Interrupted muscle sutures. Interrupted skin sutures.

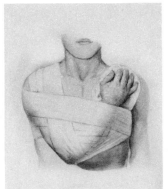

9. Method of supporting dressing and arm; Velpeau bandage.

AMPUTATION OF FOREARM

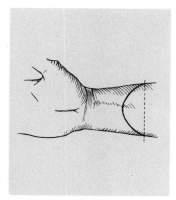

1. Surface anatomy. Anterior and posterior skin incisions.

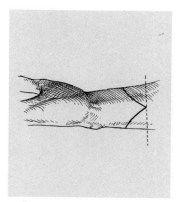

2. Lateral view. Dotted line indicates level of saw cut.

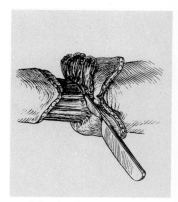

3. Muscle flap of superficial flexors to cover bone ends.

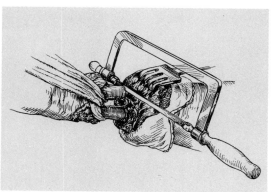

4. Circular incision carried through soft parts. Periosteum incised. Bones cut through with bone saw.

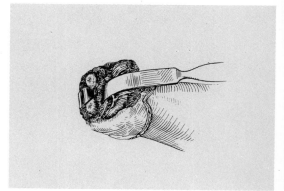

5. Muscle flap of superficial flexors retracted. Bone ends rounded and freed of periosteum.

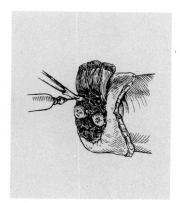

6. Large nerves pulled down, injected, and cut.

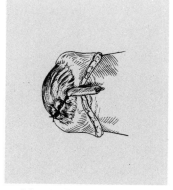

7. Muscle flap sutured to deep flexors and extensors.

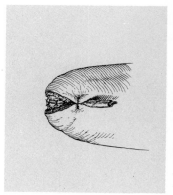

8. Interrupted sutures. Through and through rubber drain.

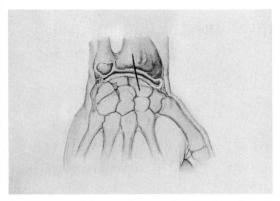

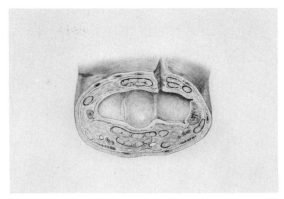

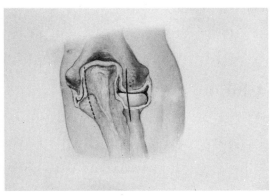

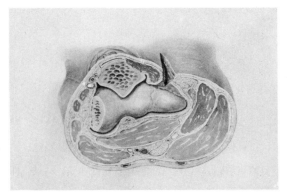

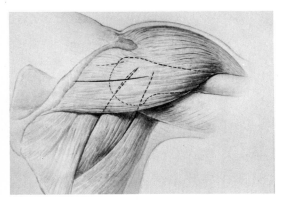

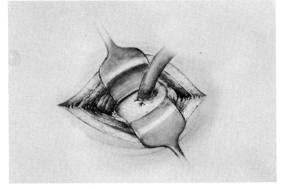

1. Diagram of bones of wrist showing location of incision for drainage of wrist joint.

2. View of wrist shows relationship of extensors and flexors to the joint space and site of incision.

3. Location of incision for drainage of elbow joint. Dotted line indicates secondary incision.

4. Sectional view of elbow joint showing relation of ulnar nerve and surrounding muscles to joint space.

5. Relation of incision for drainage of shoulder joint to underlying structures (Koenig, Stromer).

6. Arthrotomy of shoulder. Drainage tube inserted into shoulder joint and fixed with suture.

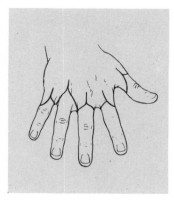

1. Surface anatomy, sites of incision for amputation of fingers.

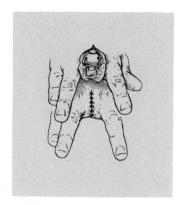

2. Metacarpophalangeal disarticulation, flap closure.

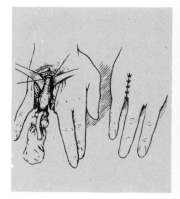

3. Amputation proximal to metacarpal head and closure.

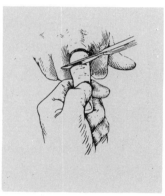

4. Interphalangeal disarticulation. Rubber band tourniquet.

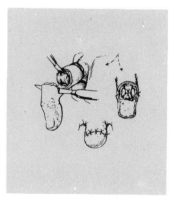

5. Tendons left long for suturing over proximal joint surface.

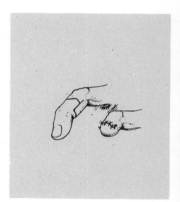

6. Amputation through phalanx. Note method of flap suture.

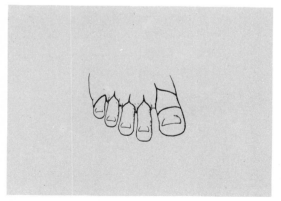

7. Surface anatomy and sites of incisions for individual amputation of the toes.

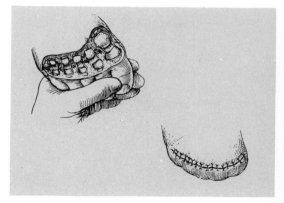

8. Metatarsophalangeal disarticulation of all toes and closure utilizing skin flap and interrupted sutures.

INCISIONS FOR DRAINAGE OF HAND INFECTIONS

(KANAVEL)

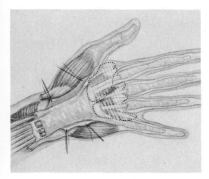

1. Relationship of palmar spaces to the tendon sheaths.

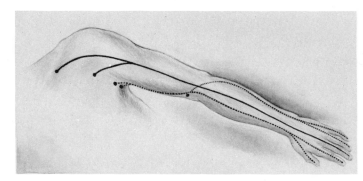

2. Entire arm showing the lymphatic drainage system for fingers, hand, forearm, upper arm, shoulder, and nodes at elbow and axilla

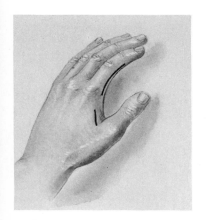

3. Incisions for tenosynovitis of index finger.

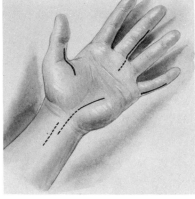

4. Incisions for tenosynovitis of flexor tendon of thumb and fingers.

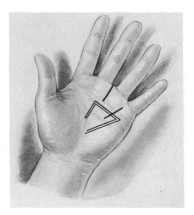

5. Incision for the drainage of mid-palmar space infection.

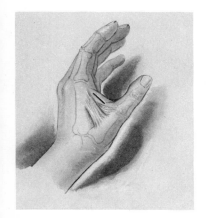

6. Incision for drainage of infection of thenar space.

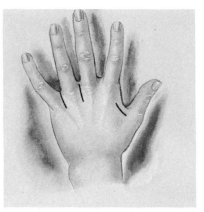

7. Accessory incisions for infections of web and thenar spaces.

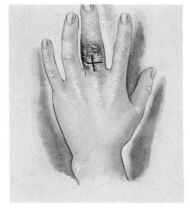

8. Location ot crucial incision for carbuncle of finger.

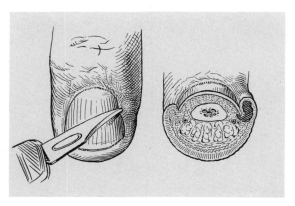

1. Incision for drainage of subepithelial abscess. Cross section shows relation of abscess to nail.

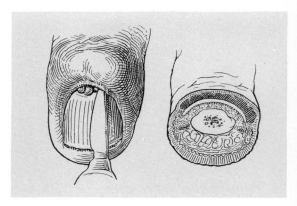

2. Incision for drainage of abscess underlying nail bed. Cross section shows extent of abscess.

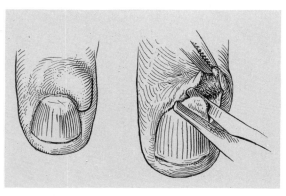

3. Fully developed paronychia. Abscess is evacuated, involved portion of base of nail removed.

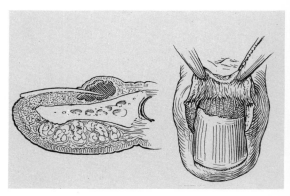

4. Fully developed subungual abscess. Bilateral incision for removal of nail root and floating portion.

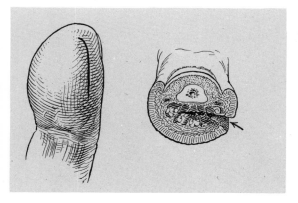

5. Location of incision for the drainage of closed space felon. Cross section shows extent of incision.

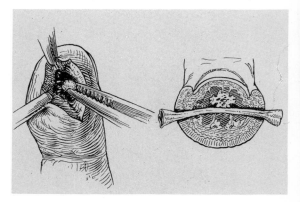

6. Bilateral incisions for felon. Removal of sequestrum not always necessary.

ARTHROPLASTY OF HIP
(SMITH-PETERSON)

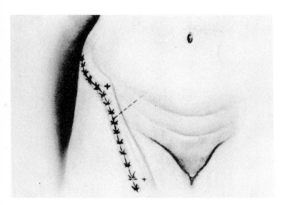

1. Surface anatomy showing line of incision and method of closure by means of interrupted silk sutures.

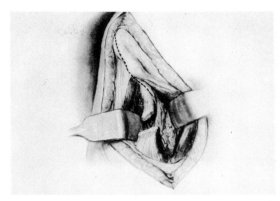

2. Sartorius muscle retracted. The rectus femoris muscle is divided.

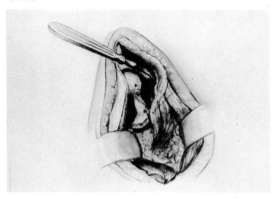

3. Muscles retracted. The periosteum is elevated and reflected from the ilium.

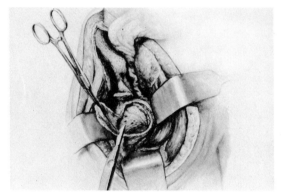

4. Method of dissecting the anterior capsule of the joint and a portion of the "Y" ligament.

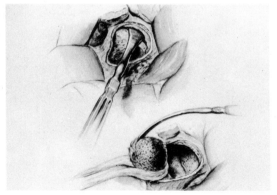

5. Head of femur freed from acetabulum, smoothed by bone rasp. Acetabulum hollowed out.

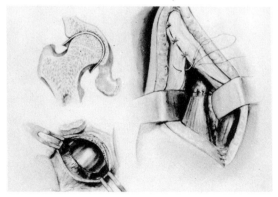

6. New head for femur made with vitallium cap. Method of closure in reconstructive layers.

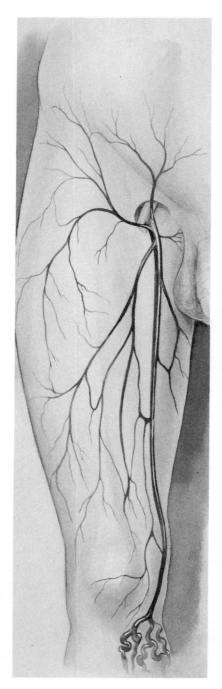

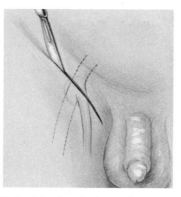

2. Incision in relation to fossa ovalis, sapheno-femoral junction.

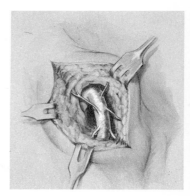

3. Incision completed. Exposure of saphenous vein and branches.

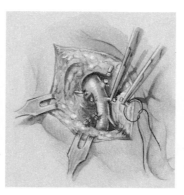

4. All branches of saphenous vein are doubly ligated and divided.

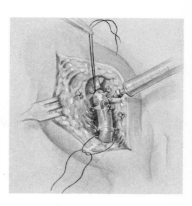

5. Long saphenous ligated. Sclerosing solution injected distally.

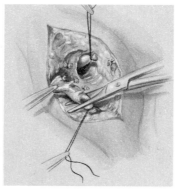

1. Sapheno-femoral junction at origin of the long saphenous vein.

6. The lower ligature is now tied and a portion of the vein excised.

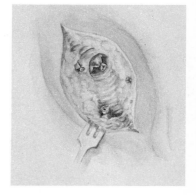

7. Operation completed. Interrupted sutures in Scarpa's fascia.

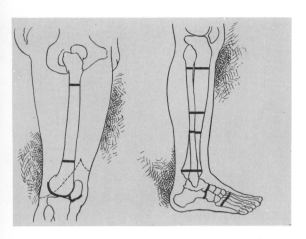

1. Anterior view of thigh and lateral view of leg showing usual sites for amputation.

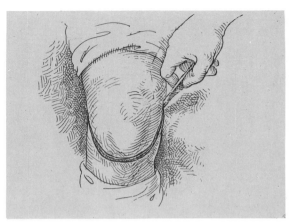

2. Amputation above knee. Incision preserves generous anterior flap of skin and subcutaneous tissue.

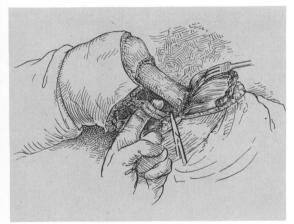

3. Incision continued through muscles to periosteum, muscles retracted. All blood vessels ligated.

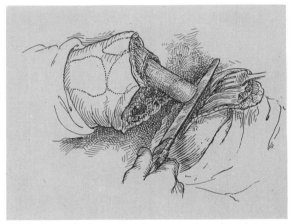

4. Amputation completed except separation of femur. Periosteum is retracted, bone divided by sawing.

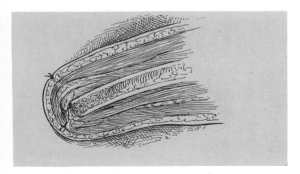

5. Severed nerves injected with alcohol. Sagittal section shows method of utilizing muscle flap to form pad.

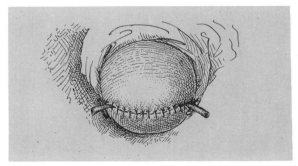

6. Amputation completed. Through and through rubber drain in place, final interrupted skin suture.

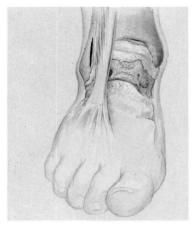

1. Incision for drainage lateral to extensor digitorum longus.

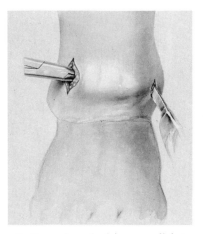

2. Secondary incision parallel to first under tip of forceps.

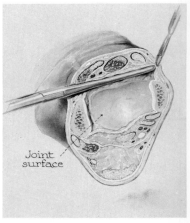

3. Joint space showing anatomical relations and position of forceps.

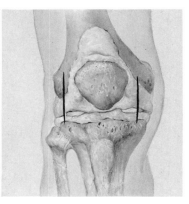

4. Bilateral incisions of knee joint on either side of patella.

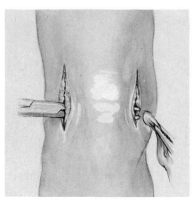

5. Trans-patella drainage for bursal infection involving joint.

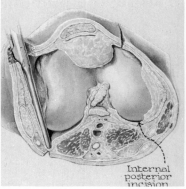

6. Cross section demonstrating bilateral anteroposterior drainage.

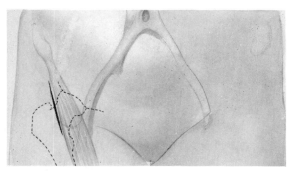

7. Diagrammatic drawing with head of femur outlined. Heavy line indicates location of incision.

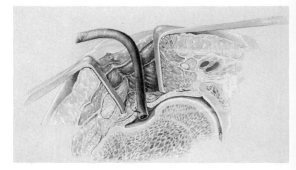

8. Sectional view showing method of insertion and attachment of drainage tube in hip joint cavity.

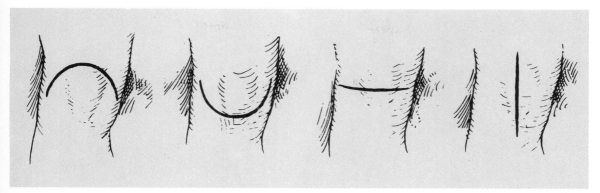

1. Surface anatomy showing four elective sites of incision for approach to the patella. Superior and inferior hemispheric incisions, horizontal and vertical incisions.

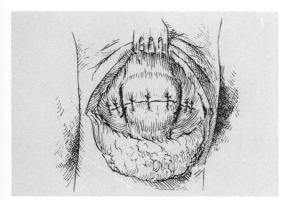

2. Method of placing deep sutures of kangaroo tendon lateral to patella, avoiding the joint cavity.

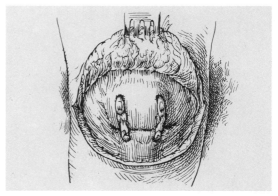

3. Method of repair with deep sutures, utilizing strips of fascia lata for suture material.

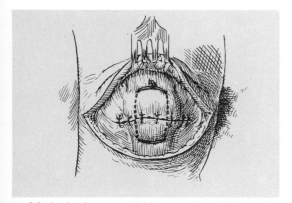

4. Method of accomplishing repair utilizing wire passed through drill holes in patella.

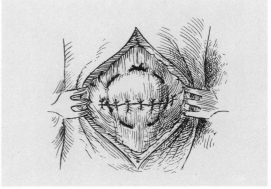

5. Method of repair utilizing circular suture of kangaroo tendon, chromic catgut, or silk.

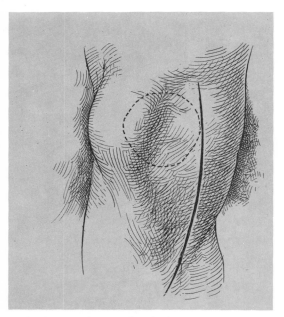

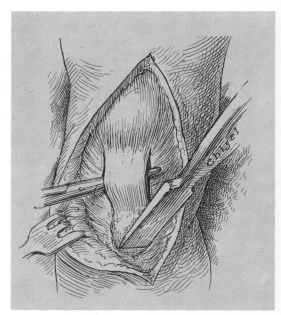

1. Surface anatomy, deformity, and line of incision. Dotted line indicates normal position of patella.

2. Patella ligament freed by sharp dissection. Tibial attachment removed with bony block by chisel.

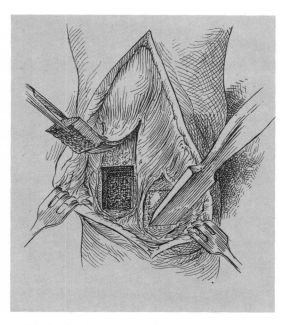

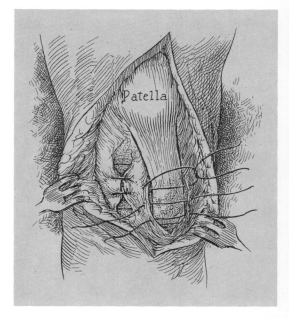

3. Block of bone with patella ligament detached. New site being prepared by chisel.

4. Initial block in new site. Second block inserted in bed of first by interrupted periosteal sutures.

BUNIONECTOMY
(MCBRIDE)

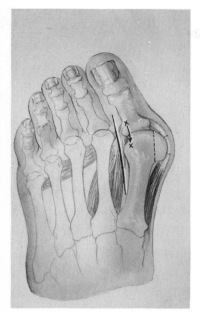

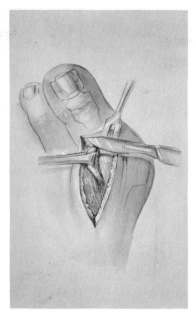

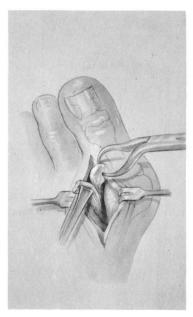

1. Incision. Dotted line indicates portion of bone to be removed.

2. Common adductor tendon severed from proximal phalanx.

•3. Removal of medial sesamoid bone. Tendon held in Allis forceps.

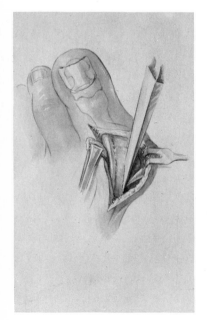

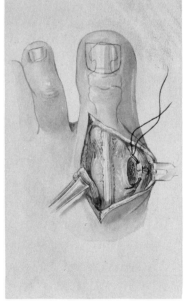

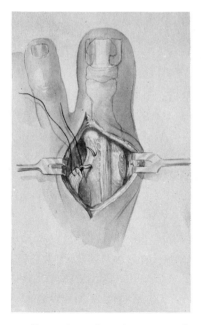

4. Method of removal of bunion by utilizing osteotome.

5. Method of shortening of abductor hallucis tendon and capsule.

6. Transplantation of common adductor tendon to first metatarsal.

BUNIONECTOMY
(KREUSCHER)

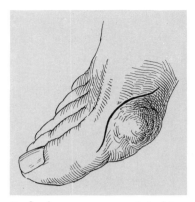

1. Surface anatomy and incision dorsal to the involved skin area.

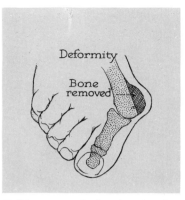

2. Diagrammatic drawing showing deformity and bone to be removed.

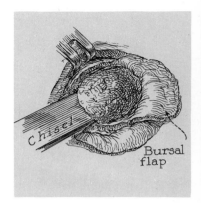

3. Skin retracted. The bursal flap has been incised and is reflected.

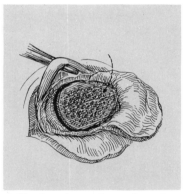

4. Tendon elevated, rough surface of bone covered with bone wax.

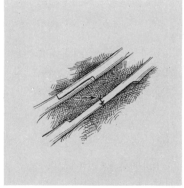

5. Extensor hallucis longus lengthened by means of "Z" tentomy.

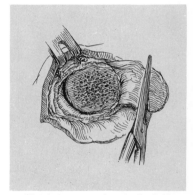

6. Tendon restored to its bed. Bursal flap trimmed to cover bone.

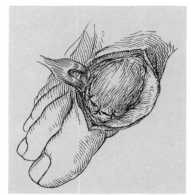

7. Trimmed bursal flap approximated by interrupted sutures.

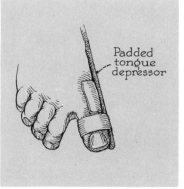

8. Initial step in dressing. Application of padded tongue depressor.

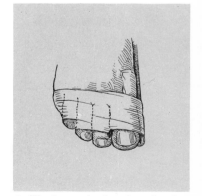

9. Final step in dressing showing means of supporting splint.

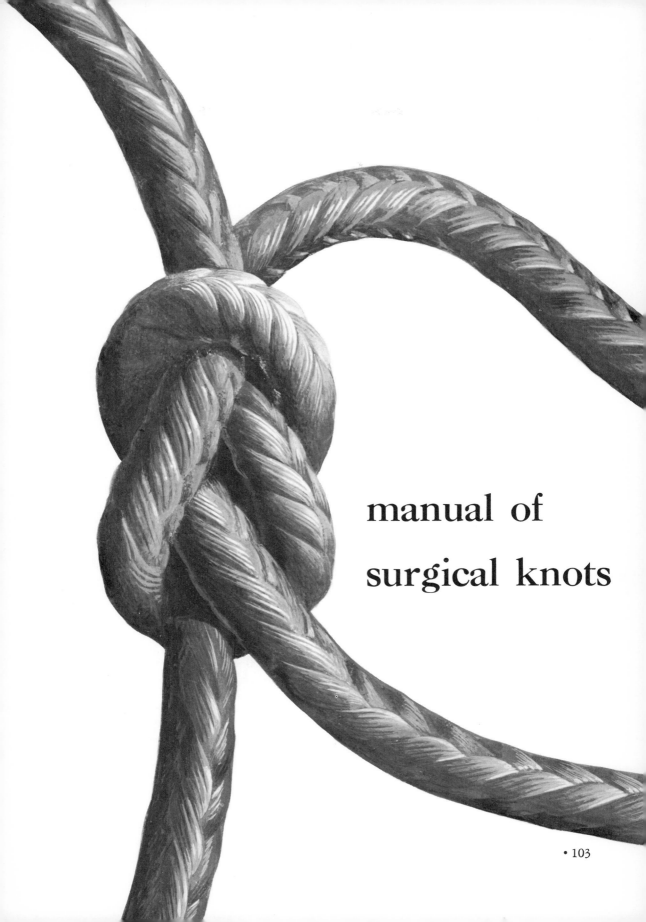

manual of
surgical knots

Dexterity and speed in tying knots correctly constitute an art which only practice can make perfect.

Of the more than 1,400 different types of knots described in The Encyclopedia of Knots only a few are used in modern surgery. But it is of paramount importance that each knot the surgeon places be perfect — that it hold with proper tension.

In the early days of surgery, materials were heavy and crude, knots bulky and inefficient. It was not unusual to place three or even four knots in the same suture "just to be sure."

Research and refinements of manufacture and sterilization have provided the surgeon with a wide choice of suture materials. The successful use of any of them is dependent upon skillful knot tying. The widespread adoption of finer gauge sutures has been accompanied by more refined suturing technics. The trend is toward simplification and standardization.

There are certain general principles which govern the tying of all knots and which apply to all kinds of suture material:

1. The completed knot must be firm, and so made that slipping is impossible. The simplest knot is the most desirable.

2. The knot must be small: to prevent an excessive amount of tissue reaction when absorbable sutures are used; to minimize foreign body reaction to non-absorbable sutures. "Whiskers" should be cut short.

3. In tying any knot, "sawing" (friction between strands) must be avoided as it weakens the integrity of the suture. Clamps and hemostats should never be placed on any portion of the suture which is to remain *in situ*.

4. Excessive tension applied by the operator will cause frequent breaking. Practice in avoiding excessive tension leads to successful use of finer gauge materials.

5. Sutures (for other than hemostatic purposes) should not be tied too tightly, as this causes tissue strangulation.

6. After the first loop is tied, it is necessary to maintain traction on one end of the strand for control to avoid loosening.

7. The perfect hemostasis demanded in modern surgery requires the use of a large number of ligatures. Extra ties do not add to the strength of a properly tied knot . . . they only contribute to its bulk.

The knots demonstrated on the following pages are those most frequently used, and are applicable to all types of surgery.

The Double Square Knot is recommended only when nylon sutures are used. Nylon is relatively inflexible and has an extremely smooth surface, making necessary this additional precaution to prevent slipping.

The Granny Knot is the only one shown which is *not recommended.* It is frequently and ill-advisedly used and is shown here only to warn against its use. It will not hold when subjected to increased pressure.

The step-by-step pictures are reproduced from actual photographs. The camera was placed behind the demonstrator so that each procedure is shown as seen by the operator. For clarity, one-half of the strand is black and the other white. In all of these demonstrations, *the black strand is initially held in the right hand.*

The student will find it helpful to practice the technics by following the successive steps shown in the photographs, using a piece of string. After he has become familiar with the various steps, he should practice them without watching his hands.

In this manner he will literally as well as figuratively be able to tie these knots "with his eyes closed." The last phase in learning is to tie the knots wearing gloves and using actual suture materials.

Knot tying is a detail in the complex art and science of surgery, but it is important and warrants thorough mastery.

good knot-tying technic

An important part of good suturing technic is correct method in knot tying.

A seesaw motion, or the sawing of one strand down over another until the knot is formed, may materially weaken sutures to the point that they may break easily when the second throw is made.

If the two ends of the suture are pulled in opposite directions with uniform rate and tension, there will be less tendency to disrupt the peripheral fibers, and the knot may be tied more securely with less possibility of breakage. This point is well-illustrated in the knot-tying pictures shown in the next section of this book.

square knot
...two-hand technic
The technic of choice when conditions permit.

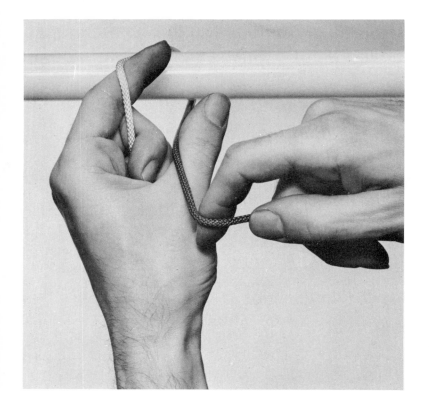

White strand placed over extended index finger of left hand acting as a bridge, and held in palm of left hand. Black strand held in right hand brought between left thumb and index finger.

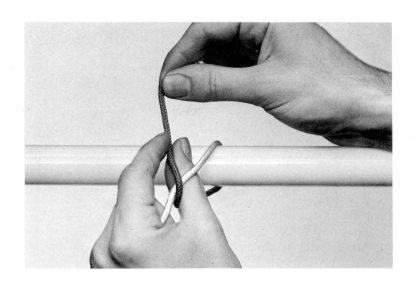

Left hand turned inward by pronation, and thumb pushed under white strand. Black strand crossed over white and caught between thumb and index finger of left hand.

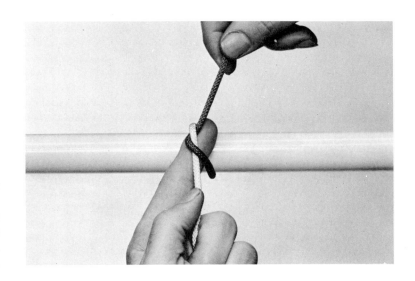

Left hand turned outward by supination with thumb and index finger still grasping black strand and pushing through the white loop. Black strand is released by left hand and grasped by right.

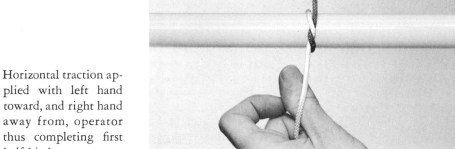

Horizontal traction applied with left hand toward, and right hand away from, operator thus completing first half hitch.

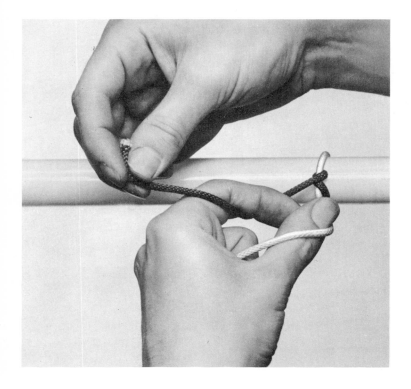

Left hand turned inward by pronation and black strand placed in angle between left thumb and index finger. Index finger is then flexed over black strand and placed beneath thumb.

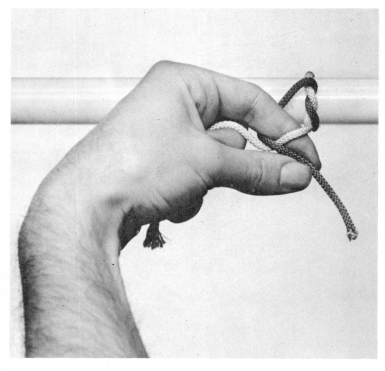

White strand slides on to index finger of left hand, black is placed over white and grasped by left index finger and thumb.

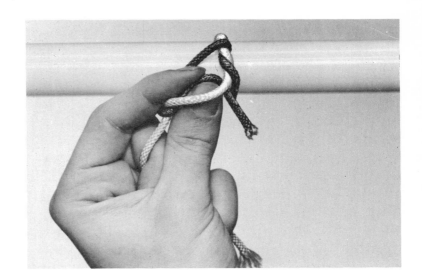

Left hand rotated inward by pronation with thumb carrying black strand through loop.

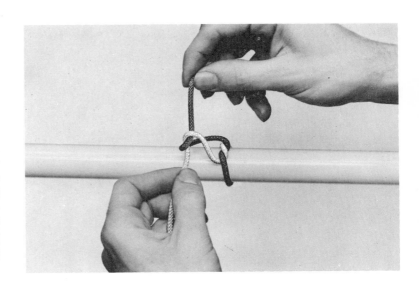

Black strand released from left index finger and grasped by right hand. Second half hitch is completed by reversing position of hands — black strand remains in right hand and white in left.

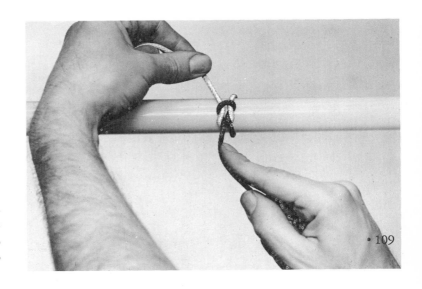

Hands in reverse position and horizontal traction applied with left hand away from, and right hand toward, operator.

square knot
...one-hand technic

The Square Knot has withstood the test of time and experience and is universally recommended. Wherever possible it is tied using the two-hand technic. On some occasions it will be found necessary to use one hand, either the left or the right.

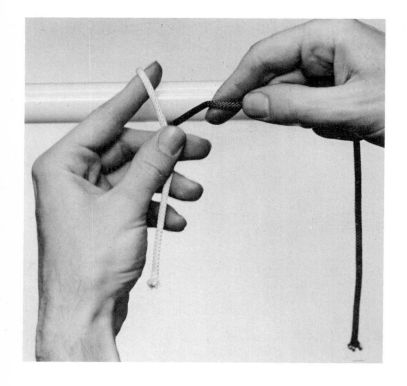

White strand held between thumb and second finger of left hand with index finger elevated as bridge. Black strand held between thumb and index finger of right hand.

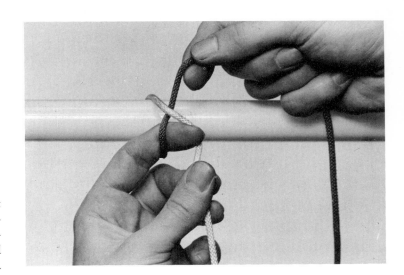

Distal phalanx of left index finger passed under black strand supported in right hand and over white strand.

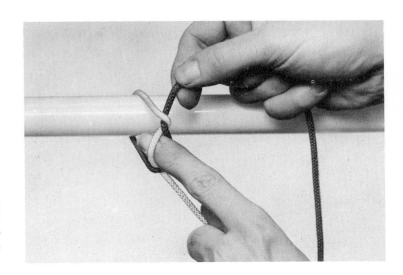

Left hand rotated inward by pronation, and white strand pulled through loop by extension of left index finger.

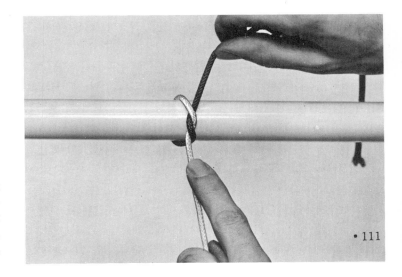

Completion of first step by traction in horizontal plane — left hand drawn toward, and right hand away, from operator.

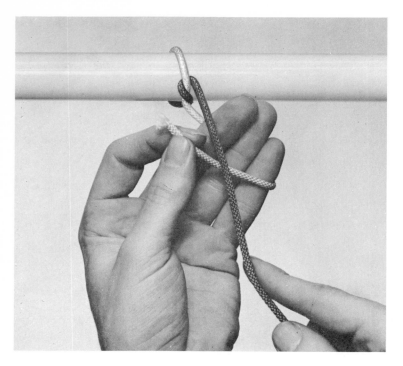

White strand looped around three fingers of left hand, and distal end held between thumb and index finger. Black strand held in right hand and brought over white strand.

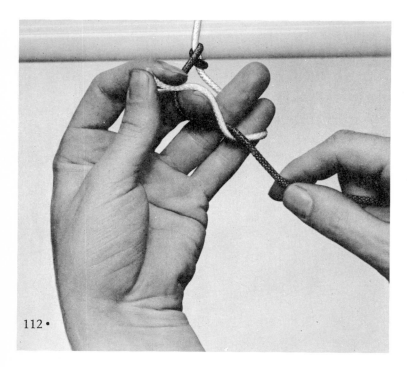

Distal phalanx of left second finger is flexed, thus pulling black strand forward and beneath white strand. Tip of second finger of left hand is extended so that white strand is brought behind it.

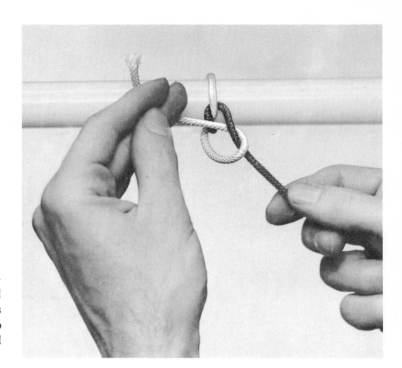

Left hand is rotated inward by pronation, and second finger of this hand extended to bring white strand through loop.

Square knot completed by horizontal traction. Left hand away from, and right hand toward, operator.

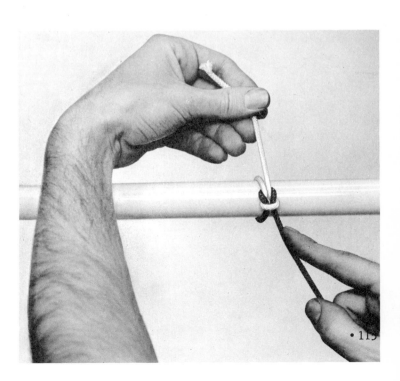

instrument tie

The Instrument Tie is useful where one or both ends are short.

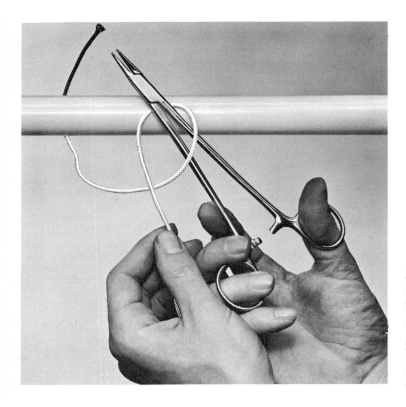

Short black strand is free, long white end held between left thumb and index finger. First loop formed by passing needle holder around white strand.

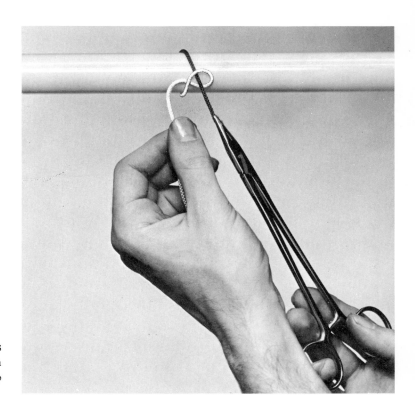

Needle holder grasps short black end which is pulled through loop toward operator.

First half hitch completed by pulling needle holder toward operator and white strand away from operator. Needle holder released.

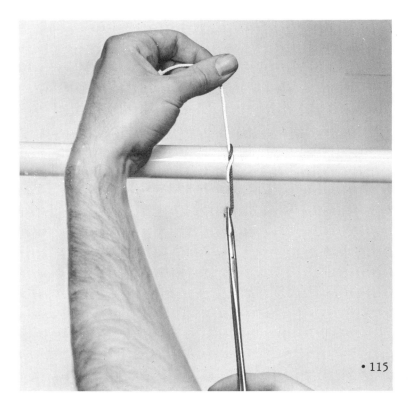

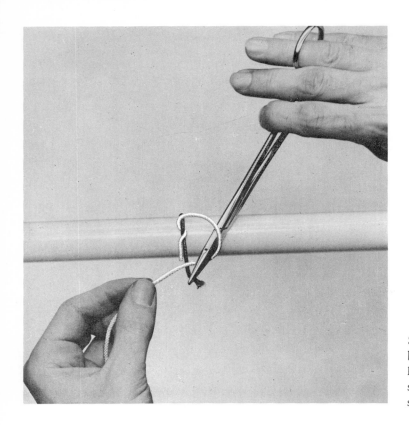

Second loop is formed by passing needle holder over white strand and grasping short black end.

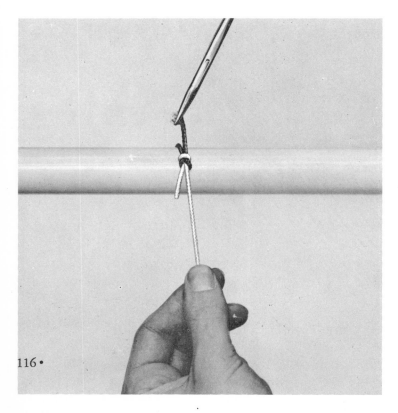

Square knot completed by traction with short end pulled away from, and long end toward, operator. (The long end may be grasped by another instrument instead of hand in all steps.)

slip knot

The Slip Knot is used at points difficult of access, such as a deep pedicle stump or for hemostasis in tonsillectomies, or where the knot must be frequently adjusted or untied.

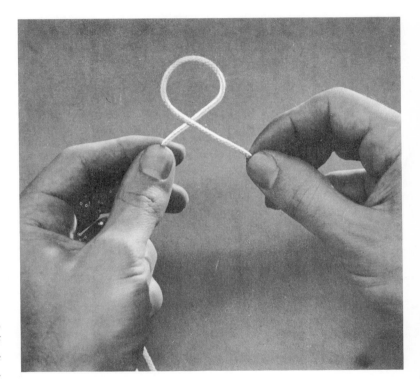

A loop is formed so that the short end of the strand held in the right hand lies on top.

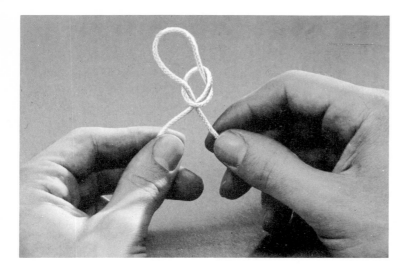

The forefinger of the right hand has pushed a small loop through the loop made in the first step. (The second loop may be pulled through the first by the left thumb and index finger if this is preferred.)

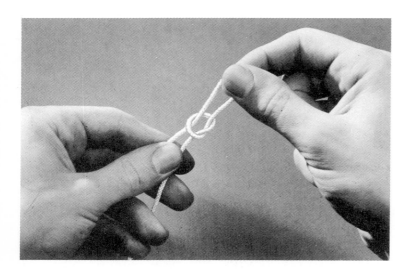

The slip knot is prepared by pulling on the loop. The short end is held by a needle holder, hemostat or other suitable instrument. The hemostat to be used on the bleeder is slipped through the loop prior to grasping the bleeder.

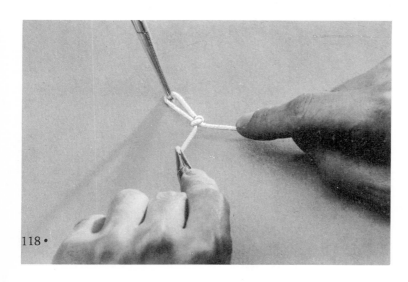

Final position before pulling long end of strand to set knot at the desired site. This knot may be secured by the addition of a square knot, if desired.

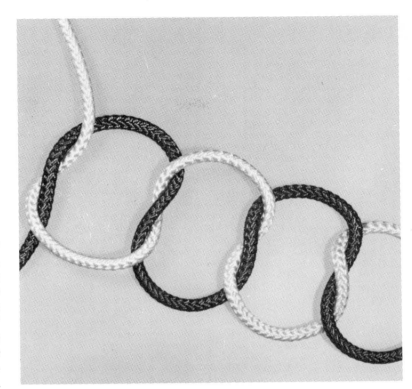

double square knot
above a Granny Knot, recommended in tying nylon sutures. The Granny Knot permits closer "pulling down" of the nylon. The Square Knots anchor and prevent any slippage of the Granny.

group of knots
commonly used, left to right: Simple Knot; Square Knot; Granny Knot (not recommended); Surgeon's or Friction Knot; Surgeon's Knot completed — a Simple Knot tied above a Friction Knot.

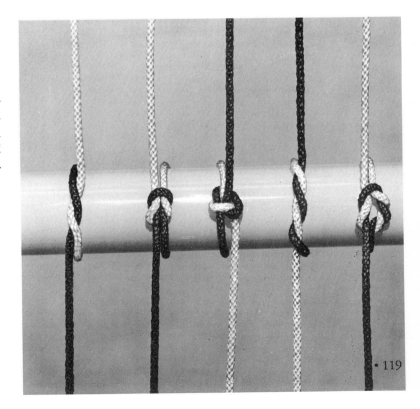

SUTURES

Suture material is divided into two general classes, Absorbable and Non-Absorbable. Absorbable Sutures are those which are absorbed or digested during the healing process by the tissues in which they are placed. Non-Absorbable Sutures are not affected by the digestive action of body fluids. They remain in the body unless they are cast off or removed.

Absorbable Sutures are made of surgical gut, except for a very minor supply of kangaroo tendon, which is occasionally used in certain work. Non-Absorbable Sutures are made chiefly of silk, MERSILENE® polyester fiber, linen, cotton, nylon, metal, horsehair and silkworm gut.

Surgical gut is the principal suture material in surgery. It is used in far greater quantity than all other suture materials combined.

The choice of the suture depends on these factors:

1. The presence or absence of infection in the operative area at the time of operation.
2. The type of tissue to be approximated.
3. The desirability of permanent support of the tissues.

Surgical gut sutures are made from the submucosa or fibrous layer of the small intestine of the sheep. Surgical gut is prepared in several sizes, and also in various types which have different time-spans of absorption in tissue.

Since surgical gut is absorbed, it is not a permanent foreign body. As absorption occurs, scar tissue develops and binds the approximated structures together.

Non-Absorbable Sutures should not be used in the presence of active infection, since bacteria become harbored in the interstices and the suture acts as a continual feeder of the infective organisms.

Non-Absorbable Sutures should be used on all large arteries, whether the field is sterile or not. Silk is preferred to surgical gut for bad traumatic wounds, after they have been completely debrided.

ETHICON **CP** surgical gut

virtually non-antigenic because it is COLLAGEN PURE

The exclusive Ethicon chemical cleaning process removes all but a trace of noncollagenous protein. This assures sutures of virtually pure collagen — and pure collagen does not produce allergic reactions. CP surgical gut is exclusive with Ethicon.

stronger because it is TRU-GAUGED

An ordinary catgut suture may vary as much as a full size in diameter at several points along its length, but Ethicon surgical gut is Tru-Gauged. The diameter is uniform along the full length of the suture strand. The tensile strength of Ethicon Tru-Gauged surgical gut far exceeds U.S.P. requirements. Thus, smaller sizes can be used with a consequent reduction of trauma.

ETHICON surgical gut ▶
has uniform diameter along full length of strand. Tensile strength exceeds U.S.P. requirements. Trauma is lessened.

ORDINARY catgut ▶
suture may vary as much as a full size in diameter at several points along its length.

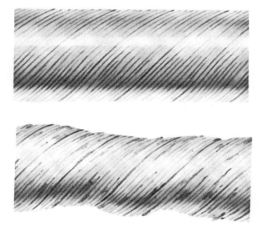

ETHICON CP
surgical gut
digests more uniformly
because it is
TRU-CHROMICIZED

Ordinary catgut is surface chromicized after the strand is spun. The chrome salts are deposited only on the outer surface of the suture. Ethicon surgical gut is Tru-Chromicized. The chrome salts are deposited on each ribbon before the strand is spun, thus assuring even distribution of chrome throughout the suture. This insures an even, dependable rate of digestion.

Ethicon processes Collagen sutures from raw sheep instestine to finished strands. *Only* Ethicon CP Surgical Gut is Collagen Pure, Tru-Gauged and Tru-Chromicized. There *is* a difference in Ethicon surgical gut.

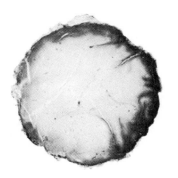

surface-chromicized gut

Microphotograph of cross section of surface-chromicized catgut suture. Intense dark areas show highly concentrated chrome in periphery of suture allowing center section to be too rapidly absorbed. Leaves highly chromicized periphery as hollow tube.

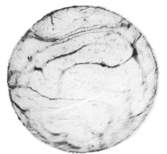

ribbon-chromicized gut

Microphotograph of cross section of ribbon-chromicized surgical gut suture shows almost even distribution of chrome throughout suture. Ribbon-chromicized surgical gut tends to digest evenly from periphery to center.

surgical needles

With the growth of surgery, there have been many types of needles introduced. It may be confusing to the embryo surgeon to pick out the proper needle for a procedure when he sees the vast number of needles available today.

Most men are able to perform any type of operation with only one or two different needles. Experience alone will tell the surgeon which is best suited for his particular needs. One caution may be stated. The needle should not be larger nor stronger than is necessary for the particular tissue in which it is used, nor for the suture which it carries.

An eyed needle has three distinctive parts: the point, the shaft, and the eye. There are four types of points: the cutting edge, the spear point or triangular, the tapering point, and the trocar point. The shaft may be either straight or curved. A curved needle is used in a region where the point may be difficult to see after the needle has passed through the tissue.

With the adoption of finer sutures, the problem of eyed needles became more important. The ordinary needle, upon insertion into tissue, pulls after it a double strand of suture which forms a larger hole through the tissue than is really necessary for the single strand of suture which follows. This added trauma may be sufficient to cause difficulties, particularly where the possibility of leakage of any fluid may occur through the suture holes.

The most recent advance in needle design is the "eyeless" needle. The suture is swaged to the needle by mechanical pressure. This is the ATRALOC® needle, which draws a single strand of suture through the tissue. Minimal damage is done to tissue by this type of needle and suture.

BASIC SURGICAL NEEDLE COMPONENTS

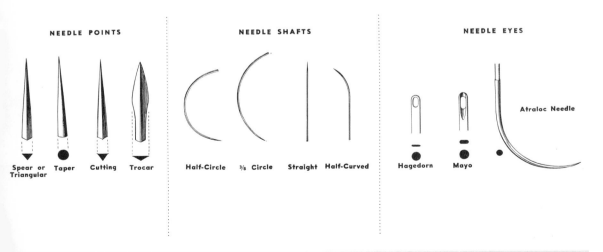

NEEDLE POINTS — Spear or Triangular, Taper, Cutting, Trocar
NEEDLE SHAFTS — Half-Circle, ⅜ Circle, Straight, Half-Curved
NEEDLE EYES — Hagedorn, Mayo, Atraloc Needle

ONLY ETHICON® MAKES

ATRALOC® SEAMLESS NEEDLES
less trauma — less tissue disruption

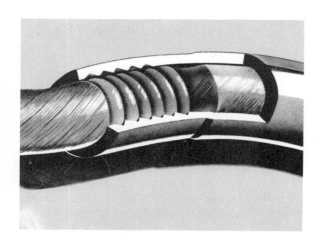

The end of each ATRALOC seamless needle is drilled and threaded, the gut clamped into place, and the needle cold-pressed.

ATRALOC seamless needles provide:

• an ideal needle-suture combination for the specific surgical need

• a new, sharp needle with each suture

• improved points — consistent sharpness — easier penetration

• longer, more useful area — needle won't turn in holder

NEW REVERSE CUTTING NEEDLES

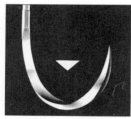

reverse cutting ATRALOC needle: cutting edge on bottom

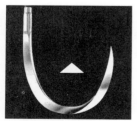

ordinary cutting needle: cutting edge on top

New reverse cutting ATRALOC needle is triangular throughout its entire length. This increases needle strength as much as 40 per cent, and greatly reduces chances of bending or breaking. Natural cutting action is assured because cutting edge is on outside of needle curve. Cutting edges extend to a point just beyond maximum width of needle. After this point, needle retains triangular shape but not the cutting edge. And since there is no change in needle shape, resistance is minimized as needle penetrates tissue.

• Less tendency to cut out of tissue

• 40% greater needle strength

• Easier penetration with less trauma

• Will not turn in needle holder

OPERATIVE PROCEDURE

INDEX

INDEX